Diagnosis and Management of Pediatric ENT Conditions

Editor

STEVEN L. GOUDY

CLINICS IN PERINATOLOGY

www.perinatology.theclinics.com

Consulting Editor
LUCKY JAIN

December 2018 • Volume 45 • Number 4

ELSEVIER

1600 John F. Kennedy Boulevard • Suite 1800 • Philadelphia, Pennsylvania, 19103-2899

http://www.theclinics.com

CLINICS IN PERINATOLOGY Volume 45, Number 4
December 2018 ISSN 0095-5108, ISBN-13: 978-0-323-64316-0

Editor: Kerry Holland
Developmental Editor: Casey Potter

Clinics in Perinatology (ISSN 0095-5108) is published quarterly by Elsevier Inc., 360 Park Avenue South, New York, NY 10010-1710. Months of issue are March, June, September, and December. Business and Editorial Offices: 1600 John F. Kennedy Blvd., Ste. 1800, Philadelphia, PA 19103-2899. Customer Service Office: 3251 Riverport Lane, Maryland Heights, MO 63043. Periodicals postage paid at New York, NY and additional mailing offices. Subscription prices are $299.00 per year (US individuals), $548.00 per year (US institutions), $351.00 per year (Canadian individuals), $670.00 per year (Canadian institutions), $433.00 per year (international individuals), $670.00 per year (international institutions), $100.00 per year (US students), and $195.00 per year (Canadian and international students). International air speed delivery is included in all Clinics subscription prices. All prices are subject to change without notice. **POSTMASTER:** Send address changes to *Clinics in Perinatology*, Elsevier Health Sciences Division, Subscription Customer Service, 3251 Riverport Lane, Maryland Heights, MO 63043. **Customer Service: Telephone: 1-800-654-2452** (U.S. and Canada); **1-314-447-8871** (outside U.S. and Canada). **Fax: 1-314-447-8029. E-mail: journalscustomerservice-usa@elsevier.com** (for print support); **journalsonlinesupport-usa@elsevier.com** (for online support).

Reprints. For copies of 100 or more, of articles in this publication, please contact the Commercial Reprints Department, Elsevier Inc., 360 Park Avenue South, New York, NY 10010-1710. Tel. 212-633-3874; Fax: 212-633-3820; E-mail: reprints@elsevier.com.

Clinics in Perinatology is also pubilshed in Spanish by McGraw-Hill Interamericana Editores S.A., P.O. Box 5-237, 06500 Mexico D.F., Mexico.

Clinics in Perinatology is covered in *MEDLINE/PubMed (Index Medicus) Current Contents, Excepta Medica, BIOSIS and ISI/BIOMED.*

Contributors

CONSULTING EDITOR

LUCKY JAIN, MD, MBA
George W. Brumley Jr Professor and Chair, Emory University School of Medicine, Department of Pediatrics, Chief Academic Officer, Children's Healthcare of Atlanta, Executive Director, Emory and Childrens Pediatric Institute, Atlanta, Georgia

EDITOR

STEVEN L. GOUDY, MD
Director of Pediatric Otolaryngology, Division of Pediatric Otolaryngology, Emory University School of Medicine, Atlanta, Georgia

AUTHORS

BRIAN T. ANDREWS, MD
Director of Cleft and Craniofacial Surgery, Associate Professor, Departments of Plastic Surgery, and Otolaryngology–Head and Neck Surgery, University of Kansas Medical Center, Kansas City, Kansas

JAY BHATT, MD
Assistant Professor, Department of Pediatric Otolaryngology, Children's Hospital Colorado, University of Colorado School of Medicine, Aurora, Colorado

SIVAKUMAR CHINNADURAI, MD, MPH
Associate Professor, Department of Otolaryngology and Facial Plastic Surgery, Children's Hospitals and Clinics of Minnesota, Minneapolis, Minnesota

KAVITA DEDHIA, MD
Department of Pediatric Otolaryngology, Emory University, Atlanta, Georgia

ELISE GRAHAM, MD
Department of Pediatric Otolaryngology, University of Utah, Salt Lake City, Utah

CHRISTOPHER HARTNICK, MD, MS
Department of Otolaryngology–Head and Neck Surgery, Massachusetts Eye and Ear Infirmary, Harvard Medical School, Boston, Massachusetts

LARRY D. HARTZELL, MD, FAAP
Associate Professor, Department of Otolaryngology–Head and Neck Surgery, Division of Pediatric Otolaryngology, University of Arkansas for Medical Sciences, Arkansas Children's Hospital, Little Rock, Arkansas

AYESHA HASAN, MD
Department of Obstetrics and Gynecology, University of Kansas Medical Center, Kansas City, Kansas

LOUIS F. INSALACO, MD
Department of Otolaryngology–Head and Neck Surgery, Boston Medical Center, Boston, Massachusetts

LUV JAVIA, MD
Assistant Professor of Clinical Otorhinolaryngology–Head and Neck Surgery, Cochlear Implant Program, Center for Pediatric Airway Disorders, Children's Hospital of Philadelphia, University of Pennsylvania Perelman School of Medicine, Philadelphia, Pennsylvania

ADAM B. JOHNSON, MD, PhD
Assistant Professor, Otolaryngology–Head and Neck Surgery, Director of Velopharyngeal Dysfunction, University of Arkansas for Medical Sciences, Little Rock, Arkansas

LAUREN A. KILPATRICK, MD
Assistant Professor, Department of Otolaryngology–Head and Neck Surgery, University of North Carolina at Chapel Hill, Chapel Hill, North Carolina

APRIL M. LANDRY, MD
Assistant Professor of Otolaryngology, Department of Otolaryngology–Head and Neck Surgery, Emory University, Atlanta, Georgia

ALEXANDER P. MARSTON, MD
Head and Neck Surgery Fellow, Division of Pediatric Otolaryngology, Department of Otolaryngology–Head and Neck Surgery, MUSC Children's Hospital, Medical University of South Carolina, Charleston, South Carolina

ALBERT PARK, MD
Department of Pediatric Otolaryngology, University of Utah, Salt Lake City, Utah

KRISHNA G. PATEL, MD, PhD
Associate Professor, Department of Otolaryngology–Head and Neck Surgery, Medical University of South Carolina, Charleston, South Carolina

EDWARD B. PENN Jr, MD
Assistant Professor, Pediatric Otolaryngologist, Department of General Surgery, Greenville Health System, Greenville ENT Associates, Greenville, South Carolina

JEREMY D. PRAGER, MD, MBA
Director, Aerodigestive Program and Associate Professor, Department of Pediatric Otolaryngology, Children's Hospital Colorado, University of Colorado School of Medicine, Aurora, Colorado

KARA PRICKETT, MD
Assistant Professor of Otolaryngology–Head and Neck Surgery, Assistant Professor of Pediatrics, Children's Healthcare of Atlanta, Emory University School of Medicine, Atlanta, Georgia

LOURDES QUINTANILLA-DIECK, MD
Assistant Professor, Department of Otolaryngology–Head and Neck Surgery, Oregon Health & Science University, Portland, Oregon

ROY RAJAN, MD
Pediatric Otolaryngologist, Lehigh Valley Health Network, Allentown, Pennsylvania

NIKHILA RAOL, MD, MPH
Department of Otolaryngology–Head and Neck Surgery, Emory University School of Medicine, Division of Pediatric Otolaryngology, Children's Healthcare of Atlanta, Atlanta, Georgia

JEFFREY RASTATTER, MD
Assistant Professor, Department of Otolaryngology–Head and Neck Surgery, Northwestern University Feinberg School of Medicine, Ann & Robert H. Lurie Children's Hospital of Chicago, Chicago, Illinois

GRESHAM T. RICHTER, MD
Professor, Otolaryngology–Head and Neck Surgery, Director of Vascular Anomalies Center, University of Arkansas for Medical Sciences, Little Rock, Arkansas

MICHAEL J. RUTTER, MD
Professor of Otolaryngology, Department of Otolaryngology–Head and Neck Surgery, University of Cincinnati, Cincinnati, Ohio

THOMAS SCHREPFER, MD
Department of Otolaryngology–Head and Neck Surgery, Emory University School of Medicine, Division of Pediatric Otolaryngology, Children's Healthcare of Atlanta, Atlanta, Georgia

ANDREW R. SCOTT, MD
Assistant Professor of Otolaryngology and Pediatrics, Departments of Pediatric Otolaryngology and Facial Plastic Surgery, Medical Director, Cleft Lip and Palate Team, Floating Hospital for Children, Tufts Medical Center, Boston, Massachusetts

DAVID ERIC TUNKEL, MD
Professor, Director of Pediatric Otolaryngology, Department of Otolaryngology–Head and Neck Surgery, Johns Hopkins School of Medicine, Baltimore, Maryland

JAMES D. VARGO, MD
Department of Plastic Surgery, University of Kansas Medical Center, Kansas City, Kansas

JONATHAN WALSH, MD
Assistant Professor, Department of Otolaryngology–Head and Neck Surgery, Johns Hopkins School of Medicine, Baltimore, Maryland

DAVID R. WHITE, MD
Director, Division of Pediatric Otolaryngology, Professor, Department of Otolaryngology–Head and Neck Surgery, Surgeon in Chief, MUSC Children's Hospital, Medical University of South Carolina, Charleston, South Carolina

MITCHELL L. WORLEY, MD
Resident Physician, Department of Otolaryngology–Head and Neck Surgery, Medical University of South Carolina, Charleston, South Carolina

TO ENROLL

To enroll in the *Clinics in Perinatology* Continuing Medical Education program, call customer service at 1-800-654-2452 or sign up online at http://www.theclinics.com/home/cme. The CME program is available to subscribers for an additional annual fee of 244.40 USD.

METHOD OF PARTICIPATION

In order to claim credit, participants must complete the following:

1. Complete enrolment as indicated above.
2. Read the activity.
3. Complete the CME Test and Evaluation. Participants must achieve a score of 70% on the test. All CME Tests and Evaluations must be completed online.

CME INQUIRIES/SPECIAL NEEDS

For all CME inquiries or special needs, please contact elsevierCME@elsevier.com.

CLINICS IN PERINATOLOGY

Foreword

Three-Dimensional Printing and Beyond: What Lies Ahead for Pediatric Otolaryngology

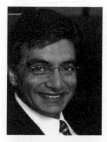

Lucky Jain, MD, MBA
Consulting Editor

In a groundbreaking surgery at Children's Healthcare of Atlanta last month, a group of surgeons, scientists, and intensivists teamed up to create and implant a personalized three-dimensional (3D)-printed device to fix the airway of a young infant who was suffering from severe tracheobronchomalacia. Over time, the infant is expected to go from having multiple near-death spells every day to a stable airway that would otherwise have been impossible to achieve.

The concept of 3D printing is not new; it arose from the automotive and aerospace industry as an additive manufacturing technique and has been more recently applied to customization of medical devices.[1,2] The field is evolving rapidly from manufacturing of static devices, such as hearing aids, amputee prosthetics, and dental appliances, to more dynamic interventions, such as the one accomplished at our center where the device is expected to conform to the rapidly growing airway (**Fig. 1**).[1] Indeed, such considerations have led to the potential for four-dimensional structures capable of engineered shape change "owing to design-influenced mechanical and degradation deformation in response to tissue growth over time."[1]

There is also the prospect of antenatal 3D printing of devices that might be needed immediately after birth. Zopf and colleagues[2] reported the first case of 3D modeling and 3D printing of complex fetal maxillofacial anatomy after prenatal ultrasound indicated potential upper airway obstruction from a midline mass of the maxilla. In a feat of bioengineering, investigators used fetal MRI and patient-specific computer-aided modeling to create the new craniofacial anatomy using a 3D printer.

Clin Perinatol 45 (2018) xv–xviii
https://doi.org/10.1016/j.clp.2018.09.002
0095-5108/18/© 2018 Published by Elsevier Inc.

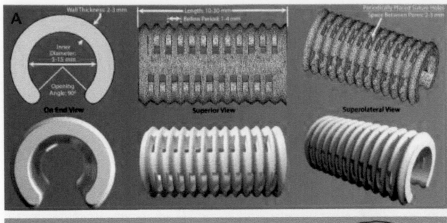

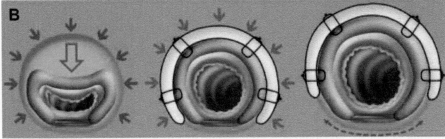

Fig. 1. Computational image-based design of 3D-printed tracheobronchial splints.(A) Stereolithography (STL) representation (top) and virtual rendering (bottom) of the tracheobronchial splint demonstrating the bounded design parameters of the device. We used a fixed open angle of 90 degrees to allow placement of the device over the airway. (B) Mechanism of action of the tracheobronchial splint in treating tracheobronchial collapse in TBM. Solid arrows denote positive intrathoracic pressure generated on expiration, hollow arrow denotes vector of tracheobronchial collapse, dashed arrow denotes vector opening wedge displacement of the tracheobronchial splint with airway growth. (C) Digital imaging and Communications in Medicine (DICOM) images of the patient's CT scan were used to generate a 3D model of the patient's airway via segmentation in Mimics. (D) Design parameters were input into MATLAB to generate an output as a series of 2D. (E) Virtual assessment of fit of tracheobronchial splint over segmented primary airway model for all patients. (F) Final 3D-printed PCL tracheobronchial splint used to treat the left bronchus of patient 2. (From Morrison RJ, Hollister SJ, Niedner MF, et al. Mitigation of tracheobronchomalacia with 3D-printed personalized medical devices in pediatric patients. Sci Transl Med 2015;7(285):285ra64; with permission.)

These are exciting developments because they carry the promise that early treatment of deformities such as tracheobronchomalacia may prevent complications often encountered with conventional treatments, such as tracheostomies and mechanical ventilation. However, further enrollment of patients under Food and Drug Administration guidelines for investigational devices to demonstrate short- and long-term safety will be required before these interventions can become standard of care.

Much progress has been made in many other areas also, including the widespread application of exit procedures,[3] early detection of hearing loss,[4] and cochlear devices[5] for hearing loss, and so forth. These and many other important topics are covered in this issue of the *Clinics in Perinatology* by Dr Goudy and his colleagues. As always, I

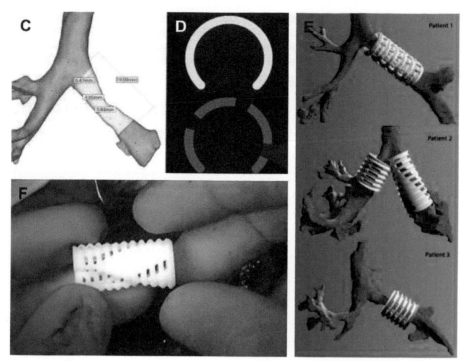

Fig. 1. *Continued*

am grateful to Kerry Holland and Casey Potter at Elsevier for their assistance with the publication of another great set of clinically relevant articles, which can come in handy for a busy clinician whenever the need arises.

Lucky Jain, MD, MBA
Emory and Childrens Pediatric Institute
Emory University School of Medicine, and
Children's Healthcare of Athlanta
1760 Haygood Drive, W409
Atlanta, GA 30322, USA

E-mail address:
ljain@emory.edu

REFERENCES

1. Morrison RJ, Hollister SJ, Niedner MF, et al. Mitigation of tracheobronchomalacia with 3D-printed personalized medical devices in pediatric patients. Sci Transl Med 2015;7(285):285ra64.

2. Zopf DA, Hollister SJ, Nelson ME, et al. Bioresorbable airway splint created with a three-dimensional printer. N Engl J Med 2013;368(21):2043–5.

3. Ryan G, Somme S, Crombleholme TM. Airway compromise in the fetus and neonate: prenatal assessment and perinatal management. Semin Fetal Neonatal Med 2016;21:230–9.

during the eighth week of gestation.[3] Failure of the larynx to undergo recanalization results in a spectrum of glottic web and laryngeal atresia.

Congenital Subglottic Stenosis

Subglottic stenosis (SGS) is a narrowing of the region extending from the infraglottic cavity to the inferior margin of the cricoid without history of intubation. Stenosis of the subglottis is defined as a diameter of 4 mm or less in full-term infants (normal diameter 4.5–5.5 mm) and 3 mm or less in premature infants (normal diameter is 3.5 mm).[4] SGS is separated into congenital or acquired in nature.

Congenital SGS is diagnosed when the stenosis is noted without a history of endotracheal intubation. If the infant has been intubated, one cannot determine if the manipulation of the airway has caused or contributed to the stenosis and it is then determined to be acquired. The true incidence of congenital stenosis is difficult to determine because many of these infants are intubated at birth. The suspected incidence of congenital SGS is 5% of all cases of SGS.[4,5] Patients with congenital SGS are at risk of developing an acquired stenosis, even when an age-appropriate endotracheal tube is used.

Congenital SGS can be due to abnormal cartilage shape or membranous thickening. The cricoid cartilage is nearly equal in diameter in the anterior-posterior and transverse dimensions. An elliptical cricoid in which the anterior-posterior diameter is greater than the transverse diameter may be found in congenital SGS. The stenosis can also be membranous where there is a circumferential, soft narrowing arising from thickening of the submucosa due to a fibrous tissue and mucous gland hyperplasia.[6,7]

Anterior Glottic Webs and Laryngeal Atresia

Anterior glottic webs and laryngeal atresia are a result of failure of the laryngeal lumen to recannulate after epithelial obliteration. These abnormities are a spectrum of disease determined by the amount of recanalization that occurred before the embryologic process was interrupted. The spectrum of anterior webs range from thin webs with little glottic involvement (**Fig. 1**) to thick webs with near complete glottic fusion and subglottic extension (**Fig. 2**).[8] If the recanalization process is interrupted early in

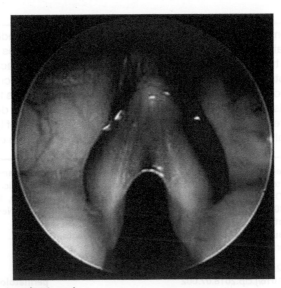

Fig. 1. Thin anterior glottic web.

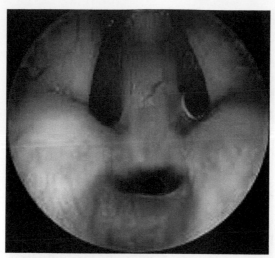

Fig. 2. Thick glottic web with subglottic extension.

its course, laryngeal atresia may occur in which there is complete obliteration of the lumen and the glottis is a fused, firm membrane and is often associated with a distal tracheoesophageal fistula. Webs are partial laryngeal atresia.

Laryngeal atresia is 1 cause of congenital high airway obstruction syndrome (CHAOS), in which lung fluid is unable to be eliminated owing to complete obstruction of the upper airway. The tracheobronchial tree and lungs fill with lung fluid and these structures subsequently dilate. CHAOS due to laryngeal atresia can be recognized prenatally owing to advances in antenatal imaging, including fetal MRI.[9] If recognized prenatally, the infant may be delivered via a planned ex utero intrapartum treatment procedure in which a tracheostomy is placed while the infant receives oxygenation via the placental circulation. If not recognized prenatally, complete laryngeal atresia will present at birth with aphonia, cyanosis, and death if a tracheostomy is not performed emergently.[10]

An association between anterior glottic webs and chromosome 22q11.2 deletion syndrome has been described by several groups.[11–14] As many as 65% of patients with anterior glottic webs have an associated 22q11.2 deletion syndrome.[11] It is recommended that all patients with anterior glottic webs should be tested by fluorescent in situ hybridization analysis, especially those with cardiac abnormalities.

Laryngeal Cleft

Laryngeal clefts are thought to be a result of the failure of the midline formation of tracheoesophageal septum. The septum forms in a caudal to cranial direction, thus the depth of the cleft is determined by the timing of the interruption in the formation of the septum. The Benjamin and Inglis system is the most commonly used classification system of laryngeal clefts.[15] The type I cleft extends to the level of the vocal cords. Type II clefts extend past the vocal cords and into the posterior cricoid cartilage (**Fig. 3**). Type III and IV clefts extend through the posterior cricoid cartilage, with the former extending into the cervical trachea and the latter into the thoracic trachea (**Fig. 4**). Management depends on the severity of the cleft. Type I clefts may be able to be managed medically with feeding therapy and thickening of feeds. Type II, III, and IV clefts typically require surgical treatment.

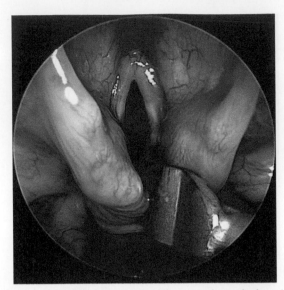

Fig. 3. Type 2 laryngeal cleft with extension into but not through the cricoid cartilage.

Laryngeal clefts are associated with other congenital abnormities in 58% to 68% of cases.[16,17] Most commonly, these anomalies occur in the digestive tract and include esophageal atresia with tracheoesophageal fistula or tracheoesophageal fistula alone. Cardiac, urogenital, and craniofacial anomalies are also commonly found in association with laryngeal clefts.[18] Laryngeal cleft have also been associated with other syndromes (**Table 1**).[1,18]

Congenital Tracheal Stenosis

Congenital tracheal stenosis is most commonly a result of complete tracheal rings in which a complete ring of tracheal cartilage forms instead of a C-shaped

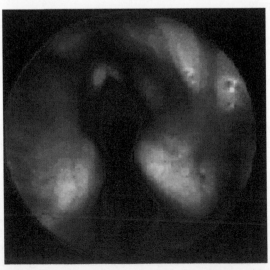

Fig. 4. Type III laryngeal cleft with extension through the cricoid and into cervical trachea.

Table 1
Syndrome associated with laryngeal clefts

CHARGE	Coloboma, heart disease, choanal atresia, growth and mental retardation, genital anomalies, ear anomalies
VACTERL or VATER	Vertebral anomalies, anal atresia, cardiac defects, tracheoesophageal fistula and/or esophageal atresia, renal or radial anomalies, and limb defects
Pallister Hall	Hypothalamic hamartoblastoma, hypopituitarism, polydactyly and syndactyly, cardiac, renal, and pulmonary abnormities
Opitz-Frias or G syndrome	Hypertelorism, hypospadias, cleft lip and palate, and other midline malformations

cartilage with a posterior membranous trachea (**Fig. 5**). The cause of this abnormality is not known but may be due to an unequal or abnormal partitioning of the foregut. Complete tracheal rings may form at any point along the tracheobronchial tree in short or long segments. Long-segment disease is typically considered to be greater than 50% of the trachea.[19,20] Narrowed segments can be as small as 1 mm and involve the length of the trachea, whereas other patients may have a short segment of mild narrowing. This is a rare disease that is estimated to affect 1 in 64,500 live births.[21] Approximately two-thirds those with complete tracheal rings will have an associated cardiac abnormality.[19,21] Pulmonary artery slings or an aberrant left pulmonary artery are the most common cardiac anomaly noted in 50% of patients with complete rings.[22] Complete rings are associated with bronchial branching abnormities, including an anomalous right upper lobe (bronchus suis), bronchial trifurcation, or a single lung.[23] If complete tracheal rings are suspected or found, echocardiograph should be performed due to the high possibility of cardiac abnormalities. Computed tomography with angiogram of the chest and reconstructions are useful to assess vascular anatomy and surgical planning. Conservative management is appropriate for patients with short-segment stenosis and the most stenotic segment is not less than 60% of normal tracheal diameter.[24]

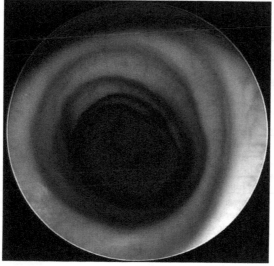

Fig. 5. Complete tracheal rings.

22. vanSon JA, Hambsch J, Haas GS, et al. Pulmonary artery sling: reimplantation versus antetracheal translocation. Ann Thorac Surg 1999 68(3):989-94.

23. Speggiorin S, Torre M, Roebuck DJ, et al. A new morphologic classification of congenital tracheobronchial stenosis. Ann Thorac Surg 2012;93(3):958-61.

24. Cheng W, Manson DE, Forte V, et al. The role of conservative management in congenital tracheal stenosis: an evidence-based long-term follow-up study. J Pediatr Surg 2006 41:1203-7.

25. Myer CM, O'Connor DM, Cotton RT. Proposed grading system for subglottic stenosis based on endotracheal tube sizing. Ann Otol Rhinol Laryngol 1994;103:319-23.

26. Wyatt ME, Hartley BE. Laryngotracheal reconstruction in congenital laryngeal webs and atresias. Otolaryngol Head Neck Surg 2005 132:232-8

27. Parkes WJ, Propst EJ. Advances in the diagnosis, management, and treatment of neonates with laryngeal disorders. Semin Fetal Neonatal Med 2016 21:270-6

28. de Alarcon A, Osborn AJ, Tabangin ME, et al. Laryngotracheal cleft repair in children with complex airway anomalies. JAMA Otolaryngol Head Neck Surg 2015;141(3):828-33.

29. Chiang T, McConnell B, Ruiz AG, et al. Surgical management of type I and II laryngeal cleft in the pediatric population. Int J Pediatr Otorhinolaryngol 2014; 78:2244-9.

30. Mathur NN, Peek GJ, Bailey M, et al. Strategies for managing type IV laryngotracheosphageal clefts at Great Ormond Street Hospital for Children. Int J Pediatr Otorhinolaryngol 2006 70:1901-10.

31. Manning PB, Rutter MJ, Lisec A, et al. One slide fits all: the versatility of slide tracheoplasty with cardiopulmonary bypass support for airway reconstruction in children. J Thorac Cardiovasc Surg 2011;141(1):155-61.

Fetal Evaluation and Airway Management

Kara Prickett, MD[a],*, Luv Javia, MD[b]

KEYWORDS

- Ex utero intrapartum treatment (EXIT) • Fetal airway obstruction
- Congenital high airway obstruction syndrome (CHAOS) • Congenital teratoma
- Lymphatic malformation • Fetal micrognathia

KEY POINTS

- Ultrasound examination and fetal MRI are the primary means of diagnosis for congenital airway obstruction. Static imaging and visualization of swallowing movements may be used to assess airway patency.
- When significant airway obstruction is expected, patients should be referred to centers capable of providing multidisciplinary maternal-fetal care and ex utero intrapartum treatment.
- Common indications for ex utero intrapartum treatment or a procedure requiring a secondary team in the operating room include head/neck teratomas, cervicofacial venolymphatic malformations, and micrognathia.
- These teams include obstetrics/maternal-fetal medicine, adult/pediatric anesthesia, pediatric otolaryngology, pediatric surgery, neonatal intensive care, ultrasonography, and operating room support staff for mother and baby.
- Equipment and detailed plans for multiple potential routes of access to the airway should be immediately available during any peripartum fetal airway intervention.

INTRODUCTION

Advances in prenatal care and imaging technology over the past 40 years have led to the consideration of the fetus as a viable, individual patient at increasingly early gestational ages. Congenital anomalies once diagnosed at birth are now routinely suspected and confirmed during the prenatal period, allowing for planning and sometimes the institution of therapy before the birth of the child. Within the realm of otolaryngology, the adoption of ex utero intrapartum treatment (EXIT) has allowed for dramatic changes in the management of anomalies causing obstruction of the fetal

Disclosure Statement: No disclosures.
[a] Department of Pediatrics, Children's Healthcare of Atlanta, Emory University School of Medicine, 1400 Tullie Road, NE, Atlanta, GA 30329, USA; [b] Cochlear Implant Program, Center for Pediatric Airway Disorders, Children's Hospital of Philadelphia, University of Pennsylvania Perelman School of Medicine, 3401 Civic Center Boulevard, Philadelphia, PA 19104, USA
* Corresponding author.
E-mail address: Kara.prickett@emory.edu

upper airway. Previously, neonates with obstructive airway pathology were born either via standard vaginal or cesarean delivery, with a limited window for airway stabilization before the onset of hypoxic injury or peripartum demise. During EXIT, the fetus is partially delivered via hysterotomy and maintained on placental support while the airway is stabilized, either through traditional laryngoscopy or bronchoscopy or surgically via retrograde intubation or tracheotomy. In the setting of pathology that prevents all access to the airway, primary resection of the obstructing mass may be performed before completion of delivery, which is also known as operation on placental support. This article reviews current and emerging methods of fetal evaluation, indications for EXIT, and provides a detailed description of the procedure and necessary personnel.

NATURE OF THE PROBLEM

Multiple case series and reports have shown favorable near-term and long-term outcomes for both the mother and child after EXIT, but the procedure involves significant risk for both patients. In the fetus, the risk for hypoxic injury and failure to establish an adequate airway remains high. The duration of available placental support is always uncertain. Large masses may require immediate complete or partial resection, leaving the fetus at risk for hemorrhage, cranial nerve palsies, or collateral damage to surrounding structures. On the maternal side, the risk for hemorrhage is a primary concern, because the placental support is maintained through use of deep anesthesia and uterine relaxation. Although a low transverse hysterotomy is preferred during EXIT, the actual site and length of the uterine incision must be adapted to the positioning of the placenta and the fetus, as well as the anomaly present. Nontraditional hysterotomy sites may place mothers at increased risk for future uterine rupture. Wound infections may also be more prevalent after EXIT as compared with standard cesarean delivery.[1]

The marshaling of resources for successful EXIT is not to be underestimated. True multidisciplinary care is a must to ensure effective surgery and resuscitation. Teams often include obstetrics, maternal-fetal medicine, pediatric otolaryngology, pediatric surgery, neonatal intensive care, ultrasonography, maternal anesthesia, pediatric anesthesia, and full operating room support staff for both the maternal and fetal teams. The sequencing of events and location of necessary supplies must be planned meticulously to ensure there are no unnecessary delays during the procedure. Planning and rehearsing of events comes at a cost of provider time spent away from other clinically productive duties. Patient selection for EXIT remains an active area of research owing to concerns about both risk minimization and appropriate stewardship of health care resources.[2]

FETAL EVALUATION
Ultrasound Examination

The American College of Obstetricians and Gynecologists' 2016 clinical management guideline details the recommended use of ultrasound examinations in pregnancy.[3] Generally, examination of the fetal presentation and number, amniotic fluid volume, placental position, fetal cardiac activity, fetal biometry (standard measurements of growth and well-being), and an anatomic survey are considered part of routine obstetric care.[3] Detailed anatomic evaluation can typically be performed between 18 and 20 weeks of gestation. Subsequent to this, limited or targeted examinations may be performed to address specific concerns or in the setting of increased risk for an anomaly. Traditional ultrasound collects information about target structures in 2 orthogonal planes, whereas 3-dimensional (3D) ultrasound examination allows for calculation of the volume of the target region and can be depicted as a 3D rendering. This examination allows for accurate characterization of the surface topography of the fetus and can clearly demonstrate both normal and abnormal anatomy.[4] Other benefits include the ability to store examination images for later active review by a radiologist and potentially greater usability for surgeons and other nonsonographers.[4] The true diagnostic superiority of 3D or 4D ultrasound examinations (which also captures movement) has yet to be established in the literature.

When a cervicofacial malformation is detected by ultrasound examination, the details contained within the examination can greatly assist in both narrowing the differential diagnosis and in planning treatment. Important ultrasonographic characteristics of fetal cervicofacial masses are shown in **Box 1**. Imaging characteristics of common obstructive pathologies are discussed in detail in their respective sections. Serial evaluation of anomalies may be required owing to significant developmental changes over the course of the second and third trimesters, as well as to ensure adequate preparation for delivery. Complete obstruction of the upper aerodigestive tract is termed congenital high airway obstruction syndrome (CHAOS) and characterized by a specific set of findings detailed in **Box 2**. Suspicion of CHAOS based on ultrasound warrants further evaluation with fetal MRI.

Fetal MRI

The first report of successful fetal MRI was published in 1983 and was performed for a patient with placenta acreta.[5] Since that time, the use of MRI has become increasingly[6] popular owing to the ability to maintain excellent soft tissue resolution at all depths of penetration and the ability to image the entire fetus at one time. There are no proven harmful effects of limited fetal exposure to the electromagnetic fields generated by MRI and no long-term adverse effects have been documented, although this aspect is less well-studied.[7,8] Gadolinium contrast is a pregnancy class C substance and is not recommended for use owing to teratogenesis and fetal growth restriction.[9] Fast-spin T2-weighted sequences are typically recommended for fetal imaging and most scans continue to be performed with 1.5 T machines. However, 3 T machines may provide better soft tissue delineation, although they are more susceptible to motion artifact.[10] Motion artifact and fetal size limit the usefulness of MRI before 20 weeks of gestation.[11] Common indications for fetal MRI are shown in **Table 1**.

The diagnostic usefulness of MRI and its correlation with postnatal diagnosis have been evaluated by multiple authors.[12] A 2015 study of MRI results after ultrasound examination found that the MRI confirmed the prior imaging findings in 89% of patients, contradicted the ultrasound imaging in 4%, and that no anomaly was found on the MRI in 7%.[13] Of the patients in this study, 28% had additional findings noted on MRI resulting in a change in diagnosis or prognosis for 20% of the patients.[13] The timing of the study remains an important consideration because some lesions are more likely to

---

Box 1
Important ultrasound descriptors of fetal cervicofacial masses

- Anterior versus posterior location

- Echogenicity of lesion

- Homogeneous versus heterogeneous echotexture

- Forced extension of the neck

- Presence of other anatomic anomalies

- Amniotic fluid index

Box 2
Ultrasound findings in congenital high airway obstruction syndrome

Polyhydramnios

Increased echogenicity of lungs

Flattened or inverted diaphragm

Distal airway dilation

Compressed heart

Ascites

---

evolve over the course of a pregnancy than others. An evaluation of airway obstruction is best done in the third trimester and may need to be repeated close to the time of delivery to ensure an accurate characterization of the degree of airway obstruction.[11] **Fig. 1** shows a third trimester fetal MRI indicative of complete tracheal obstruction in a patient who required EXIT with tracheostomy at the time of delivery.

EMERGING METHODS OF FETAL EVALUATION
Virtual Bronchoscopy

Virtual bronchoscopy allows for clear visualization of the fetal airway as a 3D model or movie based on the images taken from the MRI. The 3D modeling software allows for virtual positioning of cameras and essentially charts a course through the center of the airway model, thus allowing for confirmation of airway patency based on imaging.[14] Virtual bronchoscopy was able to successfully predict airway patency (and therefore a lack of need for EXIT) in all 4 of the fetal cases published by Werner and colleagues.[14] It remains to be seen if similar predictive accuracy can be maintained with larger, obstructive head and neck masses.

Three-Dimensional Printing of Abnormal Airway Anatomy

The advent of relatively low cost of 3D printing has allowed for modeling of complex individual anatomy for both surgical planning and educational purposes in many fields. Proof of concept for 3D printing based on fetal imaging (ultrasound examination, computed tomography scans, and MRI) was published by Werner and colleagues,[15] showing that fidelity of the fetal imaging could be maintained despite movement artifact. VanKoevering et al[16] reported the use of a 3D printed model of the upper airway in a fetus with an anterior maxillary mass to successfully predict that standard orotracheal intubation (rather than EXIT or fetal intervention) would allow access to the airway.

Table 1
Indications for high-resolution ultrasound examination and MRI

High-Resolution Ultrasound	Fetal MRI
Maternal metallic implant in the pelvis or lumbar spine	Maternal morbid obesity
Isolated ventriculomegaly	Selected brain anomalies
Facial clefts	Thoracic lesions including severe congenital diaphragmatic hernia
Limb anomalies	Soft tissue masses in the head or neck
Purely cystic lesions of the posterior neck	Ultrasound findings suggestive of congenital high airway obstruction syndrome
Screening for anomalies in high-risk patients	

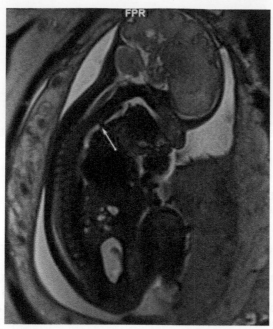

Fig. 1. T2-weighted MRI sequence with complete tracheal occlusion (*single arrow*) with fluid filling the proximal and distal airways.

Fetal Tracheoscopy

Fetal endoluminal tracheal occlusion is frequently performed in cases of severe congenital diaphragmatic hernia and involves fetoscopic placement of a detachable balloon in the trachea to prevent egress of fetal lung fluid and to stimulate lung growth. A similar technique has been reported for fetal tracheoscopy, in which a uterine trocar was placed and an exchange catheter was introduced into the airway over a flexible fetoscope allowing for both examination of the fetal airway and for the placement of a standard 2.5 mm inner diameter endotracheal tube before delivery.[17] Securing the airway before delivery allows for standard cesarean delivery, thus minimizing risk to the mother. Limitations of this technique include both the requirement for significant experience in fetal surgery and the fact that preterm delivery may be required to maintain access to the fetal mouth before descent into the maternal pelvis.[17] There are insufficient data to compare outcomes of fetal tracheoscopy with EXIT.

COMMON INDICATIONS FOR EX UTERO INTRAPARTUM TREATMENT
Oral and Cervical Teratomas

Teratomas are rare congenital malformations containing elements of endoderm, mesoderm, and ectoderm at varying levels of differentiation (**Fig. 2**). Approximately 5% to 10% of teratomas are found in the head and neck, leading to an incidence of 1:20,000 to 1:40,000 live births.[18,19] There are multiple theories of embryogenesis of teratomas, with general agreement they arise from abnormal migration or sequestration of germ cells during the fourth to fifth week of development.[18,20] Many originate in the oropharynx and nasopharynx, and are thought to be due to the proximity of all 3 germ layers at the fetal buccopharyngeal membrane. Epignathus is sometimes mentioned as a separate lesion, but represents a teratoma of the highest degree of

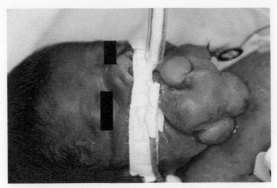

Fig. 2. Neonate with a large oral cavity congenital teratoma delivered via ex utero intrapartum treatment (EXIT). The patient's airway was intubated at the time of EXIT.

differentiation (often with recognizable internal structures or organs) classically arising from the maxilla or sphenoid.

Teratomas are typically seen without associated anomalies, so diagnostic examination should focus on local involvement or encasement of structures in the head and neck.[18] On ultrasound examination, teratomas present as heterogeneous masses with solid and cystic components in the anterior neck with extension across the midline; internal calcifications are highly specific for teratoma.[6,18] MRI typically shows a well-circumscribed, heterogeneous, and multiloculated mass with frequent involvement of the thyroid in cervical lesions.[18,21] In cases of epignathus, evaluation for intracranial extension is particularly important.[22] Approximately 20% of head and neck teratomas present with maternal polyhydramnios indicative of upper airway obstruction.[6] Owing to the firm, and often transspatial nature of the mass, a detailed delivery plan is necessary. In primarily exophytic tumors that grow out through the fetal mouth, standard cesarean delivery may be appropriate in the absence of signs of upper aerodigestive tract obstruction. For more endophytic tumors or primary cervical lesions, EXIT is frequently necessary.

Once the airway is secured, complete resection is recommended as soon as safely feasible for the neonate owing to the risk of rapid enlargement of the cystic components of untreated lesions, which can lead to mechanical obstruction or high-output heart failure (**Fig. 3**).[21] Malignancy is rare in head and neck teratomas resected in the neonatal period, but commonly seen in lesions not diagnosed until adolescence or adulthood.[6,19,20] Malignant transformation has been reported in only 9 of 220 cases in the literature and is diagnosed based on the presence of metastasis or pathologic findings consistent with undifferentiated, primitive tumor.[6,18]

Micrognathia

Fetal micrognathia (abnormal size of the mandible) may be seen with or without retrognathia (abnormal position of the mandible). When severe, micrognathia can lead to glossoptosis with resultant upper airway obstruction (**Fig. 4**). In the Pierre Robin sequence, micrognathia and glossoptosis lead to cleft palate owing to failure of fusion of the palatal shelves. More than one-half of infants with Pierre Robin sequence or nonsyndromic micrognathia experience respiratory distress after delivery and can be challenging to intubate.[23] The anomaly is also rarely seen in isolation. Up to 66% of patients with micrognathia have associated chromosomal anomalies, with commonly associated syndromes including Stickler, Nager, Treacher Collins, and

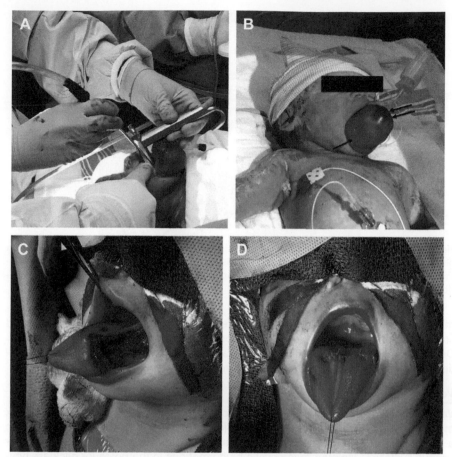

Fig. 3. (A) Distraction of the teratoma out of the mouth allowed for traditional laryngoscopy and securement of the airway with orotracheal intubation over a Hopkins rod. (B) Neonatal patient with airway secured at conclusion of the ex utero intrapartum treatment procedure. The native tongue is noted on right (*single arrow*) with a cystic teratoma displacing the tongue from left (*double arrow*). (C) The lesion was resected from the lingual and sublingual spaces on day of life 1 after the neonate was resuscitated and stabilized. Both lingual arteries and the vast majority of the native tongue were preserved. (D) Repaired tongue after tumor resection.

velocardiofacial syndromes.[23,24] A Japanese study of fetal and neonatal autopsy specimens collected over 40 years showed that 100% of patients with micrognathia had associated anomalies, including 80% with musculoskeletal abnormalities, 60% with genitourinary anomalies, and 60% with cardiovascular anomalies.[25]

Micrognathia can be objectively defined as a jaw index of lees than the 5th percentile, typically given as a value of less than 23, with 100% sensitivity and 98.7% specificity.[26] The jaw index is calculated based on measurements in 2 planes (**Box 3**) and has been shown to be more accurate than an assessment of the fetal profile.[26] Although it is an excellent predictor of micrognathia, the jaw index is not particularly specific for predicting airway obstruction owing to the micrognathia.[26] Many infants with micrognathia can be managed successfully with conservative measures such as prone positioning, alternative feeding methods, and nasal trumpets. Severe

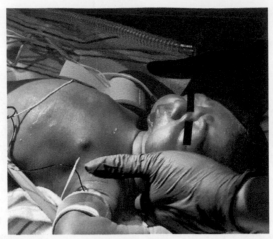

Fig. 4. Neonate delivered via a procedure requiring a secondary team in the operating room (PRESTO) with severe micrognathia and microstomia. Owing to severe obstructive breathing, patient's airway was secured with an laryngeal mask airway (LMA) followed by fiberoptic intubation through the LMA.

micrognathia and micrognathia accompanied by polyhydramnios or other ultrasound findings of upper aerodigestive obstruction are considered indications for EXIT.[26] Definitive management after initial airway stabilization may require mandibular distraction osteogenesis with or without tracheostomy.[27]

Venolymphatic Malformations

Venolymphatic malformations (VLMs) represent the most common congenital neck masses diagnosed during the fetal period (**Fig. 5**).[22] They are thought to result from a failure of the lymphatic channels to make appropriate contact with the jugular venous system.[24] Isolated macrocystic malformations in the posterior neck are typically diagnosed in the second trimester and are frequently associated with fetal aneuploidies; these lesions are commonly referred to as cystic hygromas in obstetric and older otolaryngology literature. Lesions diagnosed in the third trimester are more likely to be located in the anterior neck, are more frequently mixed microcystic and macrocystic lesions, and are more likely to intimately involve or encase surrounding structures (**Fig. 6**). They are more likely to occur as isolated anomalies. Transspatial, cystic lesions may be identified on ultrasound examination, typically with absent Doppler signal, although in more vascular lesions flow may be seen. MRI is helpful in delineating the margins of the lesion, with T2 signal predominating. Fluid–fluid levels may be present in some cysts. At times, differentiation between cystic teratoma and VLM based on imaging findings alone may be difficult.

Box 3
Calculating the jaw index

$$Jaw\ Index = \frac{Anterior - Posterior\ Diameter}{Biparietal\ Diameter} \times 100$$

Data from Paladini D, Morra T, Teodoro A, et al. Objective diagnosis of micrognathia in the fetus: the jaw index. Obstet Gynecol 1999;93(3):382–6.

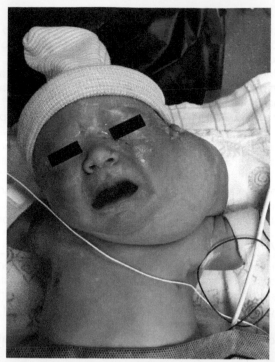

Fig. 5. Neonate delivered via a procedure requiring a secondary team in the operating room with a large cervicofacial venolymphatic malformation.

The majority of fetal lymphovascular malformations do not require intrapartum treatment. A 18-year review by Laje and colleagues[28] cited need for EXIT in only 11% of fetuses (13/112) with a prenatally diagnosed lesion. Many patients can be managed

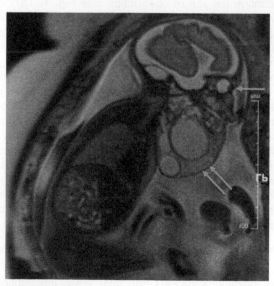

Fig. 6. Multiloculated mixed microcystic and macrocystic venolymphatic malformations involving the fetal tongue, submental space, and retropharyngeal space (*double arrow*). The fetal eye marked for reference (*single arrow*).

with orotracheal intubation with or without aspiration of macrocysts to improve access to the airway. In cases of diffuse endolaryngeal involvement, tracheotomy with retrograde intubation or formalized tracheostomy may be necessary.

Lymphatic malformations tend to be less destructive than teratomas. They are less likely to cause severe airway distortion leading to pulmonary hypoplasia or to precipitate the need for surgical resection or exploration at the time of delivery.[28] Compression of the pharyngeal and laryngeal portions of the airway is common. The postnatal course, however, tends to be more complex and prolonged. Patients with VLMs are more likely to have severe disfigurement and persistent disease than are patients with other congenital neck masses.[29] Cranial neuropathies and feeding and speech delays are also common in this group of patients, which can lead to long-term tracheostomy or gastrostomy tube dependence.[28,30] Definitive management is typically undertaken over multiple treatments with a combination of surgical excision, sclerotherapy, and the potential addition of pharmacologic adjuvants such as sildenafil or rapamycin.

Congenital High Airway Obstruction Syndrome

Owing to the high risk for fetal and perinatal mortality, the true incidence of CHAOS is unknown. It can occur in sporadic or syndromic fashion, with associated syndromes including Fraser's syndrome, Cri-du-Chat, short rib polydactyly syndrome, and velocardiofacial syndrome.[31] A single case of a father with 2 affected sons has been reported.[31]

The constellation of findings in CHAOS stems from the accumulation of fetal lung fluid in the lower airways owing to complete obstruction at the level of the trachea or larynx. This leads to expansion of the lungs with resultant compression of the heart and inversion of the diaphragm. Expansion of the lungs may impede fetal swallowing, contributing to polyhydramnios.[32] If tracheal atresia is accompanied by tracheoesophageal fistula, classic signs may not be present, because the esophagus and pharynx provide an egress route for the lung fluid. Ultrasound findings in CHAOS are shown in **Box 2**. Fetal MRI provides detailed views of the fluid column in the fetal airway and may confirm the site of obstruction (see **Fig. 1**). Laryngeal atresia and tracheal obstruction produce similar imaging findings, but likely have different etiologies. Laryngeal atresia is thought to result from a failure of recanalization of the trachea during development, whereas tracheal obstruction likely results from abnormalities of foregut segmentation.[33]

Once the diagnosis is confirmed, referral to a center versed in fetal intervention or EXIT is essential. Serial amnioreductions may be needed to prevent preterm delivery. During successful EXIT, tracheotomy or a procedure to remove the obstructing lesion can be performed in a controlled fashion (**Fig. 7**). Fetal intervention may be considered in cases of thin, membranous airway obstruction or in severe maternal polyhydramnios. Should the patient present without a prenatal diagnosis, rapid tracheotomy is the only treatment option. Even when an appropriate prenatal diagnosis is made, the risk of fetal demise remains high owing to poor lung function, other coincident anomalies, and the risk for preterm birth. Long-term management in CHAOS and laryngeal atresia typically requires cricotracheal resection or segmental tracheal resection with or without laryngotracheal reconstruction, depending on the site of obstruction.

Rare Causes of Airway Obstruction and Other Indications for Ex Utero Intrapartum Treatment

Multiple other rare indications for EXIT and fetal airway intervention have been reported as isolated cases or in very small series. Bronchogenic cysts, enteric duplication cysts, thymic cysts, hemangioma, and fetal goiter have all been successfully

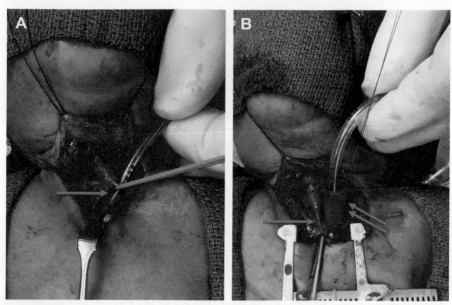

Fig. 7. (*A*) Complete tracheal atresia with a cord of tissue connecting the proximal and distal segments (*single arrow*). (*B*) A dilated distal airway is shown with an endotracheal tube in place (*double arrow*).

managed in EXIT-to-airway situations.[29,34] Cystic pulmonary airway malformations and congenital cystic adenomatoid malformations are more commonly managed with fetal intervention, such as fetal thoracoabdominal shunting, but have also been successfully treated with an EXIT-to-resection strategy.[33–35] Neuroblastoma is one of the few malignant diagnoses to be considered in obstructive fetal neck masses.[29] The use of EXIT as a bridge to other thoracic, cardiac, and abdominal procedures has been described in case reports and small series. Larger fetuses with high-risk congenital diaphragmatic hernias or thoracic lesions have been managed successfully using placement of extracorporeal membrane oxygenation catheters while on placental support (EXIT-to-extracorporeal membrane oxygenation), thus allowing for postnatal imaging and stabilization before definitive surgical resection. EXIT-to-extracorporeal membrane oxygenation management for severe congenital diaphragmatic hernia has not yet been shown to be superior to traditional management, but remains an area of active study.[36]

TIMING OF FETAL INTERVENTION

The diagnosis of potentially obstructing lesions in the fetal head and neck may occur as early as the detailed anatomy scan typically performed at 18 to 20 weeks of gestation, or may occur later in pregnancy if there is a discordance between fundal height and gestational age or if abnormal amniotic fluid indices are noted. Once diagnosed, any lesion impacting the fetal airway should be reviewed at a center with access to multidisciplinary maternal-fetal care and EXIT procedures. Owing to the presence of other anomalies and the risk for premature delivery associated with polyhydramnios, patient selection and timing of intervention remain active areas of discussion. Serial amnioreduction may be used as a method to control polyhydramnios, but its effectiveness has not been studied in randomized, controlled trials.[37] Evidence for the use of amnioreduction in singleton pregnancies is limited and generally of low quality, but suggests that risk to the fetus may be more closely related to the underlying fetal anomalies than the fluid volume or procedural intervention.[38] There is general agreement that planned EXIT before term is preferable to an emergent delivery later in gestation.[39]

Fetal hydrops is considered a strong indication for intervention, even in the preterm fetus. Nonimmune hydrops is defined as fluid accumulation in 2 or more sites, which include the fetal scalp and skin, the pleural space, the abdominal cavity (ascites), and the placenta, and may be associated with intrauterine demise in more than 90% of fetuses.[40,41] Hydrops may develop in patients with large neck masses owing to increased cardiovascular demand or arteriovenous shunting within the mass, which leads to high-output cardiac failure. If hydrops develops before 28 weeks of gestation, fetal intervention may be considered; if the fetus has matured beyond 28 weeks of gestation, delivery and definitive management are preferred.[41]

In the fetus without hydrops, serial ultrasound examinations as the pregnancy progresses to term are used to guide timing of intervention. Complex lesions may require reimaging with MRI close to the time of delivery to guide management decisions. The presence of polyhydramnios, the nature of the mass (infiltrative vs exophytic), the diagnosis, and the degree of oropharyngeal or cervical airway obstruction are all considered. Lazar and colleagues[42] attempted to quantify the degree of anatomic disruption of normal upper airway anatomy with the tracheoesophageal displacement index, which measures the degree of displacement of the trachea and esophagus from its normal location in 2 planes. They found that a tracheoesophageal displacement index of greater than 12 was highly correlated with a complicated airway at EXIT, as was the diagnosis of teratoma and the presence of polyhydramnios.[41,43] Maternal health is the other key driver of decisions regarding timing of intervention. In all maternal-fetal cases, the mother remains the primary patient, and uncontrolled maternal clinical deterioration or preterm labor should be considered indications to move toward delivery.

EX UTERO INTRAPARTUM TREATMENT PROCEDURE
Preparation

An experienced multidisciplinary team is the cornerstone for performing successful EXIT procedures in a safe manner for both the mother and fetus. This team can include maternal-fetal medicine specialists, anesthesiologists, pediatric surgeons, pediatric otolaryngologists, neonatologists, fetal cardiologists, and a specially trained group of operating room nurses and support personnel. Preoperative planning with team meetings is vital to proper planning. A variety of airway equipment is assembled in an attempt to anticipate any foreseeable airway intervention. This equipment all needs to be sterile and includes infant laryngoscopes (0, 1, and 2 Miller blades), 2.5- and 3.0-mm rigid ventilating bronchoscopes, a 2.2-mm flexible bronchoscope, cuffless endotracheal tubes, 2.5- and 3.0-mm neonatal uncuffed tracheostomy tubes, a tracheostomy surgical instrument tray, and sterile Mapleson circuit.

The EXIT procedure requires the treatment of 2 patients simultaneously, the mother and the fetus/neonate. This situation is unique, because optimizing the environment for the needs of the fetus may be at odds with the best interests of the mother. Specifically, general anesthetics such as desflurane are used to relax the uterus maximally to optimize uteroplacental gas exchange for the benefit of the fetus. These anesthetic agents can cause hypotension that may require intravenous (IV) fluids and vasopressor administration to the mother. Maternal blood pressure and cardiac output must be kept high enough to ensure sufficient placental-fetal perfusion. Interestingly, whereas in EXIT procedures uterine hypotonia is needed, in cesarean sections uterine contraction is essential to prevent maternal hemorrhage. Average maternal blood loss with cesarean deliveries can be 500 to 600 mL, whereas EXIT procedures can average maternal blood losses of greater than 1000 mL.[44,45]

In addition to the usual intraoperative monitoring, standard practice at our institution includes the placement of a urinary catheter to monitor urine output, endotracheal intubation of the mother, 2 large-bore peripheral IV lines, invasive arterial blood pressure monitoring, and an epidural catheter for the management of postoperative maternal pain.[46]

Procedure

After mapping out the placental location with an ultrasound examination and performing the hysterotomy, the fetal head, neck, and upper chest with arm is delivered, keeping the rest of the fetus within the uterus to provide uterine volume and keep the fetus warm. Warm lactated Ringer solution is continuously infused into the uterine cavity to maintain adequate uterine volume and prevent compression of the umbilical cord.[28] A pulse oximeter (wrapped in aluminum foil and a Tegaderm; 3M, St. Paul, MN) and a 24-gauge IV catheter are placed.[47] Although fetal anesthesia is accomplished through the placenta, this medication is augmented with an opioid like fentanyl and a muscle relaxant like vecuronium. Fetal vital signs are closely monitored.

Next, the fetal airway must be secured. Direct laryngoscopy is first attempted to see if the larynx can be exposed and, if so, the fetus is intubated. Standard neck extension maneuvers can help to improve exposure and suction should be available immediately. The team must keep in mind that a large tumor or malformation may need to be manipulated externally to decompress pressure on the airway or to move the airway into a more favorable position that can be seen and intubated. Intubation adjuncts such as stylettes may be helpful. Consideration can also be made for passing a needle into a large VLM to decompress a large cyst and thus relieve pressure on the airway. Large oral tumors can be partially resected to provide access to the airway, saving definitive resection for after delivery.[48]

If direct laryngoscopy is not successful in securing the airway, rigid bronchoscopy can be performed to help secure the airway. A guidewire or an intubating bougie can be fed through the bronchoscope and into the airway, which can be used to advance an endotracheal tube into position. Alternatively, an endotracheal tube can be loaded onto a rigid Hopkins rod telescope (Karl Storz, Tuttlingen, Germany). This device may be used to visualize the tracheal airway directly during bronchoscopy and then the endotracheal tube is advanced into position under direct visualization. Another possible strategy for securing the airway is fiberoptic intubation, using an endotracheal tube loaded onto a 2.2-mm fiberoptic scope.

If all anterograde efforts fail to secure the fetal airway, a tracheotomy can be performed. Anteriorly based tumors or malformations can make this procedure very challenging and thus preoperative imaging and planning are important.[49] Surgical neck exploration, tumor resection, or tumor debulking may need to be done to access the airway. Retrograde intubation technique can be useful, especially in the case of large cervical teratomas.[28,47] This process involves exposing the trachea, performing a tracheotomy incision, and feeding a 4F to 8F nasogastric tube retrograde up to the mouth. The endotracheal tube is then sutured to the tip of the nasogastric tube and the endotracheal tube is fed into the tracheal airway as the nasogastric tube is pulled back out of the tracheotomy. After positioning the endotracheal tube, the tracheotomy incision is sutured closed. If retrograde intubation is not possible, the tracheostomy may be formalized. Modern EXIT procedure protocols can allow for more than 90 minutes of time for establishing a secure airway.[28]

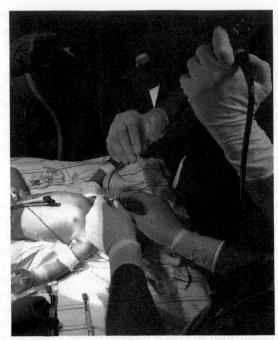

Fig. 9. Neonate with micrognathia and evidence of respiratory distress at time of a procedure requiring a secondary team in the operating room delivery. The patient successfully underwent a fiberoptic intubation through a laryngeal mask airway after the administration of ketamine and dexmedetomidine.

communication between all the parties involved with clear delineation of responsibilities and needs. Moreover, there should be a well-defined plan of how the various teams involved are activated/notified if the mother should develop early labor. We have faced instances in which the needs of mother in preterm labor so occupied the obstetrics team that timely notification of the pediatric anesthesia and pediatric otolaryngology teams was not prioritized. Comprehensive airway management at delivery may require setup of a significant amount of equipment, which can be difficult in an urgent or emergent setting.

The formation of the fetal treatment team can be another challenge. In our institutions, the core teams present at EXIT or PRESTO deliveries include neonatology, pediatric anesthesia, pediatric otolaryngology, nursing, and respiratory teams, in addition to team members devoted to maternal care. Pediatric surgeons attend deliveries when mediastinal access to the airway may be needed. There has been resistance to having pediatric anesthesia resources at the delivery, but we feel that this is a vital component of the team. First, the otolaryngologist and anesthesiologist are often working together in the operating room on babies and children with difficult airways. This mutual experience allows for an understanding of each other's needs in difficult airway situations, including depth of anesthesia needed to manipulate a neonatal airway, need to prevent apnea, and a common understanding of airway equipment used by each team. Moreover, pediatric anesthesiologists have more experience with medications such as ketamine and dexmedetomidine, which allow for sedation without apnea. This combination allows for the neonate to continue breathing efforts without fighting against resuscitation efforts. Anecdotally, as soon as these medications are delivered, we often see the neonatal oxygen saturation and other vital signs improve. Until a difficult airway is secured, we feel that it is important to avoid apnea, because the patient's breathing efforts, albeit potentially obstructive, may be the one thing allowing for at least some ventilation.

With the multidisciplinary teams needed for EXIT and PRESTO, there also comes the issue of crowd control at the delivery. Often, these deliveries are done at academic centers where there are a myriad of health care learners present. It is important to make sure that the crowding does not inhibit or compromise the care of the patients. Before each delivery, we have all the participants do a huddle, where individuals introduce themselves and their roles. Then, the group discusses specific concerns regarding the neonate, roles/expectations of the different teams, and summarizes the airway techniques that may be used.

Owing to the needs of the neonate, there may need to be a deviation from the delivery preferences of mother or her physicians. Specifically, the obstetrics teams often would prefer the mother deliver via an induced or natural vaginal delivery. This option is not optimal for the child with potential airway obstruction, because the PRESTO airway team may not be readily available when the neonate actually is born and the time to mobilize and set up such a team could compromise safety for the child, especially during the night or on the weekend. We advocate for a scheduled cesarean delivery such that the teams can be ready and set up.

Future directions include delineating better criteria regarding when an EXIT should be done versus when a PRESTO delivery can be done. Improvements in fetal imaging will help better delineate which method of delivery is most appropriate. Virtual imaging and airway modeling may allow for different methods of airway access to be trialed before actual delivery. As fetoscopic techniques mature, management of lesions before delivery may become a more viable option. Even at experienced centers, multidisciplinary care, thoughtful planning, and clear communication remain keys to success.

Best Practices

What is the current practice?

- Many patients with suspicion of fetal airway anomalies are referred to specialty centers for prenatal evaluation and planned EXIT or PRESTO delivery.

- For patients without access to prenatal specialty care, delivery with emergent airway management may be needed.

What changes in current practice are likely to improve outcomes?

- Improved diagnostic accuracy for airway lesions that develop later in gestation.

- Appropriate patient selection for EXIT and PRESTO deliveries.

- Advances in fetal care and prenatal intervention.

Is there a clinical algorithm?

There are no current evidence-based clinical algorithms for fetal care and EXIT procedures. Recommendations are based on expert consensus and published case series.
1. Suspicion for airway obstruction noted on routine ultrasound examination.
2. Confirmation of findings with high-resolution ultrasound examination or fetal MRI.
3. Multidisciplinary evaluation including maternal-fetal medicine, pediatric otolaryngology, neonatology, and other necessary specialists.
4. Counseling of family on risks and benefits of procedure with discussion of expected outcomes for mother and child.
5. Detailed coordination and planning if EXIT or PRESTO delivery is needed.

6. Close monitoring of pregnancy so plans may be adjusted if there are signs of preterm labor or fetal distress.
7. Delivery via cesarean section under general anesthesia with airway stabilization while the fetus remains on placental support.

Summary statement

The EXIT procedure allows for planned fetal airway stabilization on placental support, dramatically decreasing the incidence of hypoxic injury or peripartum demise related to airway obstruction. Coordinated, multidisciplinary care is necessary to ensure the safe treatment of both the mother and child.

Abbreviations: EXIT, ex utero intrapartum treatment; PRESTO, procedure requiring a secondary team in the operating room.

REFERENCES

1. Noah MM, Norton ME, Sandberg P, et al. Short-term maternal outcomes that are associated with the EXIT procedure, as compared with cesarean delivery. Am J Obstet Gynecol 2002;186(4):773–7.
2. Preciado DA, Rutter MJ, Greenberg JM, et al. Intrapartum management of severe fetal airway obstruction. J Otolaryngol 2004;33(5):283–8.
3. Committee on Practice Bulletins—Obstetrics and the American Institute of Ultrasound in Medicine. Practice bulletin No. 175: ultrasound in pregnancy. Obstet Gynecol 2016;128(6):e241–56.
4. Merz E, Abramowicz JS. 3D/4D ultrasound in prenatal diagnosis: is it time for routine use? Clin Obstet Gynecol 2012;55(1):336–51.
5. Smith FW, Adam AH, Phillips WD. NMR imaging in pregnancy. Lancet 1983; 1(8314–5):61–2.
6. Kerner B, Flaum E, Mathews H, et al. Cervical teratoma: prenatal diagnosis and long-term follow-up. Prenat Diagn 1998;18(1):51–9.
7. Schwartz JL, Crooks LE. NMR imaging produces no observable mutations or cytotoxicity in mammalian cells. AJR Am J Roentgenol 1982;139(3):583–5.
8. Baker PN, Johnson IR, Harvey PR, et al. A three-year follow-up of children imaged in utero with echo-planar magnetic resonance. Am J Obstet Gynecol 1994;170(1 Pt 1):32–3.
9. Sundgren PC, Leander P. Is administration of gadolinium-based contrast media to pregnant women and small children justified? J Magn Reson Imaging 2011; 34(4):750–7.
10. Wataganara T, Ebrashy A, Aliyu LD, et al. Fetal magnetic resonance imaging and ultrasound. J Perinat Med 2016;44(5):533–42.
11. Levine D. Timing of MRI in pregnancy, repeat exams, access, and physician qualifications. Semin Perinatol 2013;37(5):340–4.
12. Kathary N, Bulas DI, Newman KD, et al. MRI imaging of fetal neck masses with airway compromise: utility in delivery planning. Pediatr Radiol 2001;31(10): 727–31.
13. Verburg B, Fink AM, Reidy K, et al. The contribution of MRI after fetal anomalies have been diagnosed by ultrasound: correlation with postnatal outcomes. Fetal Diagn Ther 2015;38(3):186–94.
14. Werner H, Lopes dos Santos JR, Fontes R, et al. Virtual bronchoscopy for evaluating cervical tumors of the fetus. Ultrasound Obstet Gynecol 2013;41(1):90–4.
15. Werner H, dos Santos JR, Fontes R, et al. Additive manufacturing models of fetuses built from three-dimensional ultrasound, magnetic resonance imaging

and computed tomography scan data. Ultrasound Obstet Gynecol 2010;36(3): 355–61.

16. VanKoevering KK, Morrison RJ, Prabhu SP, et al. Antenatal three-dimensional printing of aberrant facial anatomy. Pediatrics 2015;136(5):e1382–5.

17. Cruz-Martinez R, Moreno-Alvarez O, Garcia M, et al. Fetal endoscopic tracheal intubation: a new fetoscopic procedure to ensure extrauterine tracheal permeability in a case with congenital cervical teratoma. Fetal Diagn Ther 2015;38(2): 154–8.

18. Kadlub N, Touma J, Leboulanger N, et al. Head and neck teratoma: from diagnosis to treatment. J Craniomaxillofac Surg 2014;42(8):1598–603.

19. April MM, Ward RF, Garelick JM. Diagnosis, management, and follow-up of congenital head and neck teratomas. Laryngoscope 1998;108(9):1398–401.

20. Kountakis SE, Minotti AM, Maillard A, et al. Teratomas of the head and neck. Am J Otolaryngol 1994;15(4):292–6.

21. Brodsky JR, Irace AL, Didas A, et al. Teratoma of the neonatal head and neck: a 41-year experience. Int J Pediatr Otorhinolaryngol 2017;97:66–71.

22. Tonni G, Granese R, Martins Santana EF, et al. Prenatally diagnosed fetal tumors of the head and neck: a systematic review with antenatal and postnatal outcomes over the past 20 years. J Perinat Med 2017;45(2):149–65.

23. Morris LM, Lim FY, Elluru RG, et al. Severe micrognathia: indications for EXIT-to-Airway. Fetal Diagn Ther 2009;26(3):162–6.

24. Mirsky DM, Shekdar KV, Bilaniuk LT. Fetal MRI: head and neck. Magn Reson Imaging Clin N Am 2012;20(3):605–18.

25. Akimoto N, Ikeda T, Satow Y, et al. Craniofacial and oral malformations in an autopsy population of Japanese human fetuses and newborns. J Craniofac Genet Dev Biol Suppl 1986;2:213–33.

26. Paladini D, Morra T, Teodoro A, et al. Objective diagnosis of micrognathia in the fetus: the jaw index. Obstet Gynecol 1999;93(3):382–6.

27. Costello BJ, Hueser T, Mandell D, et al. Syndromic micrognathia and peri-natal management with the ex-utero intra-partum treatment (EXIT) procedure. Int J Oral Maxillofac Surg 2010;39(7):725–8.

28. Laje P, Peranteau WH, Hedrick HL, et al. Ex utero intrapartum treatment (EXIT) in the management of cervical lymphatic malformation. J Pediatr Surg 2015;50(2):311–4.

29. Olutoye OO, Olutoye OA. EXIT procedure for fetal neck masses. Curr Opin Pediatr 2012;24(3):386–93.

30. Kamil D, Tepelmann J, Berg C, et al. Spectrum and outcome of prenatally diagnosed fetal tumors. Ultrasound Obstet Gynecol 2008;31(3):296–302.

31. Vanhaesebrouck P, De Coen K, Defoort P, et al. Evidence for autosomal dominant inheritance in prenatally diagnosed CHAOS. Eur J Pediatr 2006;165(10):706–8.

32. Hedrick MH, Ferro MM, Filly RA, et al. Congenital high airway obstruction syndrome (CHAOS): a potential for perinatal intervention. J Pediatr Surg 1994; 29(2):271–4.

33. Ryan G, Somme S, Crombleholme TM. Airway compromise in the fetus and neonate: prenatal assessment and perinatal management. Semin Fetal Neonatal Med 2016;21(4):230–9.

34. Marwan A, Crombleholme TM. The EXIT procedure: principles, pitfalls, and progress. Semin Pediatr Surg 2006;15(2):107–15.

35. MacKenzie TC, Crombleholme TM, Flake AW. The ex-utero intrapartum treatment. Curr Opin Pediatr 2002;14(4):453–8.

36. Shieh HF, Wilson JM, Sheils CA, et al. Does the ex utero intrapartum treatment to extracorporeal membrane oxygenation procedure change morbidity outcomes

for high-risk congenital diaphragmatic hernia survivors? J Pediatr Surg 2017; 52(1):22–5.

37. Harman CR. Amniotic fluid abnormalities. Semin Perinatol 2008;32(4):288–94.
38. Dickinson JE, Tjioe YY, Jude E, et al. Amnioreduction in the management of poly-hydramnios complicating singleton pregnancies. Am J Obstet Gynecol 2014; 211(4):434 e1-7.
39. Bouchard S, Johnson MP, Flake AW, et al. The EXIT procedure: experience and outcome in 31 cases. J Pediatr Surg 2002;37(3):418–26.
40. Ozgunen FT, Güleç ÜK, Evrüke İC, et al. Fetal oropharyngeal and neck tumors: determination of the need for ex-utero intrapartum treatment procedure. Balkan Med J 2015;32(2):221–5.
41. Hirose S, Sydorak RM, Tsao K, et al. Spectrum of intrapartum management strategies for giant fetal cervical teratoma. J Pediatr Surg 2003;38(3):446–50 [discussion: 446–50].
42. Lazar DA, Cassady CI, Olutoye OO, et al. Tracheoesophageal displacement index and predictors of airway obstruction for fetuses with neck masses. J Pediatr Surg 2012;47(1):46–50.
43. Steigman SA, Nemes L, Barnewolt CE, et al. Differential risk for neonatal surgical airway intervention in prenatally diagnosed neck masses. J Pediatr Surg 2009; 44(1):76–9.
44. Butwick A, Aleshi P, Yamout I. Obstetric hemorrhage during an EXIT procedure for severe fetal airway obstruction. Can J Anaesth 2009;56(6):437–42.
45. Zamora IJ, Ethun CG, Evans LM, et al. Maternal morbidity and reproductive outcomes related to fetal surgery. J Pediatr Surg 2013;48(5):951–5.
46. Lin EE, Moldenhauer JS, Tran KM, et al. Anesthetic management of 65 cases of ex utero intrapartum therapy: a 13-year single-center experience. Anesth Analg 2016;123(2):411–7.
47. Laje P, Johnson MP, Howell LJ, et al. Ex utero intrapartum treatment in the management of giant cervical teratomas. J Pediatr Surg 2012;47(6):1208–16.
48. Laje P, Howell LJ, Johnson MP, et al. Perinatal management of congenital oropharyngeal tumors: the ex utero intrapartum treatment (EXIT) approach. J Pediatr Surg 2013;48(10):2005–10.
49. Hubbard AM, Crombleholme TM, Adzick NS. Prenatal MRI evaluation of giant neck masses in preparation for the fetal exit procedure. Am J Perinatol 1998; 15(4):253–7.

Hearing Loss and Failed Newborn Hearing Screen

Kavita Dedhia, MD[a],*, Elise Graham, MD[b], Albert Park, MD[b]

KEYWORDS

- Sensorineural hearing loss • Newborn hearing screening
- Congenital cytomegalovirus • Otitis media with effusion • Auditory neuropathy

KEY POINTS

- The Newborn Hearing Screen protocol includes a hearing screen by 1 month of age.
- A congenital cytomegalovirus screening should be done before 3 weeks of age if the Newborn Hearing Screen is failed.
- A diagnostic hearing test should be done in those who failed the hearing screen by 3 months of age.
- Early intervention is important for infants diagnosed with hearing loss by 6 months of age.
- Delayed diagnosis and intervention for hearing loss can lead to poor speech and language outcomes.

INTRODUCTION

Hearing loss is the most common congenital defect and affects approximately 3 of every 1000 newborns. The introduction of universal newborn hearing screening (UNHS) in the United States has improved timely hearing loss detection, which in turn has led to earlier speech and language intervention, hearing aid fitting, and cochlear implantation.[1–5] During this period of unprecedented hearing screening, there has been a revolution in the discovery of genes found to be associated with pediatric hearing loss. More than 50% of prelingual deafness cases are genetic, and more than 90 genes have been implicated in nonsyndromic hearing loss. The advent of targeted genomic enrichment and massive parallel sequencing has made multigene panels and more comprehensive genetic testing feasible.[6–9] In addition, congenital cytomegalovirus (cCMV) is being recognized as an important cause of pediatric hearing loss. Antiviral therapy may improve hearing and neurocognitive outcomes in severely CMV-affected infants and these promising results have provided an impetus

[a] Department of Pediatric Otolaryngology, Emory University, 2015 Uppergate Drive, Atlanta, GA 30324, USA; [b] Department of Pediatric Otolaryngology, University of Utah, 100 North Mario Capercchi Drive, Salt Lake City, UT 84113, USA
* Corresponding author.
E-mail address: kavi.dedhia@emory.edu

Clin Perinatol 45 (2018) 629–643
https://doi.org/10.1016/j.clp.2018.07.004   **perinatology.theclinics.com**
0095-5108/18/© 2018 Elsevier Inc. All rights reserved.

although this response may be more consistent at 28 to 29 weeks. Evoked responses are present at 27 to 29 weeks, although a strong stimulus is required, with slow rates of stimulus presentation. Full cochlear maturity is achieved a few weeks before term birth.[36] Given the time course for the development of the auditory system, it is important to consider gestational age when interpreting the ABR results.[37] Delayed maturation of the auditory pathway in premature infants may lead to abnormal ABR results, which may improve with time in this population.[38–42] It is important to consider obtaining repeat evaluations in this population.

Furthermore, consideration should be given to children born at home because they may not have the same tracking system as at the hospital. There are few data regarding the number of newborns after homebirth who receive NHS and the number of lost to follow-up. Usually, this group is not evaluated in the follow-up data. The group at Utah has been tracking this population for the past several years. In 2015, 86% of infants born at home received newborn hearing screening. This finding is a significant improvement from 2005 when only one-third of this population was screened for hearing loss. The Early Detection and Hearing Intervention (EDHI) program in Utah attributes this improvement to increasing education and greater access to screening equipment.

AMERICAN ACADEMY OF PEDIATRICS AND CENTERS FOR DISEASE CONTROL AND PREVENTION GUIDELINES FOR THE REEVALUATION OF HIGH-RISK CHILDREN WHO PASS NEWBORN HEARING SCREENING

Children who have passed their NHS but who have additional risk factors for hearing loss should undergo a repeat hearing evaluation by the age of 24 to 30 months (**Box 1**).[16] This guideline was set in place to identify children who are at risk to develop

---

Box 1
Risk indicators associated with permanent congenital, delayed-onset, or progressive hearing loss in childhood

Caregiver concern regarding, speech, language or developmental delay

Family history of permanent childhood hearing loss

NICU duration of stay of greater than 5 days

NICU for any period of time with the following: extracorporeal membrane oxygenation, assisted ventilation, exposure to ototoxic medications, or loop diuretics, and hyperbilirubinemia requiring exchange transfusion

In utero infections: toxoplasmosis, rubella, cytomegalovirus, herpes, syphilis

Craniofacial anomalies including those that involve the pinna, ear canal, ear tags, ear pits, and temporal bone anomalies

Physical findings associated with a syndrome known to include sensorineural or permanent conductive hearing loss

Syndrome associated with hearing loss

Neurodegenerative disorders

Culture-positive postnatal infections associated with sensorineural hearing loss (meningitis)

Head trauma, especially basal skull/temporal bone fracture requiring hospitalization

Chemotherapy

Abbreviation: NICU, neonatal intensive care unit.

---

delayed-onset postnatal hearing loss and those children with mild hearing loss who may have been missed on the newborn hearing screening. With this second screen, children would be identified before preschool and intervention could be started earlier to improve speech and language outcomes.[16]

Additionally, all children should be monitored during their well check visits at 9, 18, 24, and 30 months of age for middle ear disease, auditory and speech skills, and developmental milestones using the validated global screening tool recommended by the American Academy of Pediatrics. If there is parent or physician concern for hearing, speech, or language delay, the assessment should be performed earlier.[16]

Diagnostic Auditory Brainstem Response or Auditory Steady-State Response

The ABR is considered the gold standard diagnostic test for newborn hearing assessment. This test does require specialized training for both administration and interpretation, a considerable amount of time and additional resources for cases that require sedation. An attractive but less studied alternative to the ABR is auditory steady state response (ASSR) testing. ASSR may provide some advantages over ABR in that a statistical algorithm determines whether a response is present. Thus, most of the subjectivity needed for conventional methods of reading waveforms from broad-spectrum click or tone-burst stimuli is removed.[43] Recent studies comparing ASSR with ABR, however, have reported varying results. A 2016 study by Celik and colleagues[44] demonstrated a moderate threshold correlation between the ASSR and the ABR, where previous studies have shown a stronger correlation. At this point, the ASSR is not recommended as an alternative to the ABR, but may serve as a complementary test.

EVALUATION OF THE INFANT WHO FAILS THE NEWBORN HEARING SCREEN

In 2014, we proposed that CMV testing should be performed first for the child who presents with idiopathic SNHL.[45] When early CMV testing was performed in a large group of children who presented with SNHL, we noted a high yield, low cost, and avoidance of additional genetic testing or temporal bone imaging for the cCMV-positive group. If CMV testing is negative in the presence of a failed newborn hearing screen, additional testing is recommended based on the laterality of the hearing loss. For bilateral hearing loss, genetic testing is recommended. For unilateral or asymmetric hearing loss, imaging is recommended. A proposed flow sheet is presented in **Fig. 1** from an international pediatric otolaryngology group consensus recommendation published 2 years ago.[46]

Interpretation of Middle Ear Fluid in the Infant

Otitis media with effusion (OME) is a common finding in infants who fail their newborn hearing screening. Several large studies have reported that between 55% and 65% of infants who failed their NHS have OME.[47,48] OME may be reassuring to the primary care provider and family, because this finding may explain why the newborn failed the hearing screening test. In fact, Boudewyns and colleagues[48] noted that none of the 64 infants with OME and a failed NHS were found to have an underlying SNHL. In contrast, Boone and colleagues[47] detected an underlying SNHL in 11% of infants who presented with a failed newborn hearing screening and middle ear fluid.

Boone and colleagues' finding is higher than that reported by Boedewyns and colleagues, but does appropriately illustrate the importance of considering SNHL in these more hearing screening tests, a CMV assay is run before the child is 3 weeks of age. This approach was first described on a large scale by Stehel and colleagues.[62] They initiated this protocol at one of the busiest birthing hospitals in the United States in which a urine CMV culture or polymerase chain reaction assay was performed for any infant who did not pass an aABR study before discharge. Over a 5-year period, 24 of 473 infants (5%) who failed the inpatient newborn hearing screen and underwent CMV screening tested positive for cCMV. The significance of this finding is that these children would have been unlikely to have been diagnosed otherwise. The identification of these children provides an opportunity for audiologic surveillance to detect late-onset hearing deficits that could affect language acquisition and educational achievement.

In July 2013, the first statewide hearing targeted CMV program was initiated in Utah. We identified 14 cCMV-infected infants in the 2 years after the implementation of this approach.[63] We also reported on the unexpected finding that infants who failed their newborn hearing screening and underwent CMV screening improved their time to diagnose hearing loss. The percentage of all referred infants undergoing diagnostic hearing evaluation by 3 months of age increased from 56% 2 years before the mandate to 77% at 2 years after the mandate. The ramifications of this result are that this CMV screening approach benefited the time to diagnose hearing loss in all infants who fail their newborn hearing screen.

We have also started to implement targeted CMV screening based on presentation for possible symptomatic disease. A recent study reported better hearing and neurocognitive outcomes in infants with symptomatic cCMV treated with valgancyclovir.[64] This finding provides a strong rationale to diagnose symptomatic cCMV-infected infants as soon as possible. We have recommended CMV testing in infants less than 3 weeks of age who present with abnormal head size, intrauterine growth retardation, hepatosplenomegaly, elevated transaminases, petechiae, unexplained thrombocytopenia, or intracranial abnormalities. We have diagnosed 8 cCMV-infected infants screened in just 3 NICUs over the past 2 years.

Universal CMV screening has also been advocated in a recent consensus statement.[65] Fowler and colleagues[66] reported that a targeted CMV approach that tests newborns who fail their NHS identified the majority of infants with CMV-related SNHL at birth. However, 43% of the infants with CMV-related SNHL in the neonatal period and cCMV infants who are at risk for late-onset SNHL were not identified by NHS. Such early progressive loss is surprising, because an earlier study by Fowler and colleagues[67] reported a much later onset of progressive loss. Unfortunately, the type of NHS and subsequent behavioral hearing testing were not presented. Hopefully, a subsequent publication or additional studies will provide insight into the advantages and limitations of a hearing targeted CMV approach.

Universal CMV screening would be a major undertaking. Approximately 4 million newborns would need to be screened if a nationwide universal CMV approach were introduced. Currently there are no data to support early identification of CMV-infected normal hearing infants, especially because most will never develop SNHL.[68] For those who develop late-onset SNHL, additional studies need to be performed to determine whether early diagnosis would improve their speech and language outcomes.

Imaging

Obtaining imaging is an integral component of the hearing loss workup, because abnormalities have been identified in 27.4% to 39.0%.[6,69,70] We recommend obtaining imaging as the initial diagnostic test in the following instances: asymmetric, unilateral, or progressive SNHL, or auditory neuropathy. The most common radiographic abnormality is an enlarged vestibular aqueduct, which is associated with progressive SNHL and Pendred syndrome. The most common radiographic abnormality for unilateral SNHL is a hypoplastic cochlear nerve.

High-resolution computed tomography (HRCT) scans have historically been considered the investigation of choice for patients with hearing loss.[71] HRCT is able to identify cochlear dysplasia, labyrinthine ossification, dehiscence of the semicircular canals, and position of the tegmen and sigmoid sinus, as well as the course of the facial nerve and dehiscence.[72,73] However, approximately 57% of soft tissue abnormalities of the inner ear may not by identified with a CT scan.[74] This result is especially important when determining the presence or absence of the cochlear nerve.[73] Clemmens and colleagues[75] have reported that 26% of children with unilateral SNHL will have a hypoplastic cochlear nerve. The cochlear nerve is abnormally small if, on a sagittal projection of the internal auditory nerve bundle, the nerve is found to have a smaller diameter than the facial nerve or if the color of the nerve is a lighter gray than the facial nerve[75] Although stenosis of the cochlear nerve canal, which can be measured on HRCT, is used to indirectly predict cochlear nerve aplasia, it may not be a sensitive enough modality.[7,72] A bony cochlear nerve canal that is less than 4.7 mm does strongly predict cochlear hypoplasia.

In our opinion, MRI temporal bone imaging has become our imaging modality of choice. Although imaging takes longer and is more expensive than HRCT, the ability to measure the cochlear nerve diameter and the avoidance of ionizing radiation are compelling reasons for ordering this study. The diameter of the cochlear nerve is especially important when a cochlear implant is being considered. An absent cochlear nerve is a relative contraindication for cochlear implantation because a functioning cochlear nerve is critical for a successful outcome. Children with hypoplastic cochlear nerves will have poorer hearing outcomes compared with those with normal sized nerves.[76]

Genetic Testing

Genetic factors account for approximately 50% of congenital hearing loss, and of these, nonsyndromic causes represent 70%. In syndromic hearing loss, there are associated anomalies that provide clues to the etiology of hearing loss. For example, in Usher syndrome, an autosomal-recessive cause of hearing loss and the most common cause of concurrent deafness and blindness, one might expect to see retinitis pigmentosa in addition to SNHL. There are more than 500 syndromes that have been associated with hearing loss and far more nonsyndromic genetic causes, making genetic screening for all possible causes of hearing loss very difficult.

An important question to address is the appropriate timing and patient population who require genetic screening and which genes should be included in the screen. Expert opinion suggests that patients with a defined intrauterine exposure or insult such as a TORCH infection do not require routine genetic screening.[77] Likewise, those patients with obvious sequelae of syndromes should undergo genetic testing targeted toward the most likely syndrome rather than a broad screen. Those patients in whom other testing is recommended are those with congenital bilateral hearing loss without an obvious external cause.

The most common cause of genetic hearing loss is a mutation in the gene coding for Connexin 26, a protein responsible for maintaining endolymphatic potential through potassium ion transport. The gene locus coding for this protein is the gap

13. Vohr B, Jodoin-Krauzyk J, Tucker R, et al. Early language outcomes of early-identified infants with permanent hearing loss at 12 to 16 months of age. Pediatrics 2008;122:535–44.
14. Kennedy CR, McCann DC, Campbell MJ, et al. Language ability after early detection of permanent childhood hearing impairment. N Engl J Med 2006;354:2131–41.
15. Pimperton H, Blythe H, Kreppner J, et al. The impact of universal newborn hearing screening on long-term literacy outcomes: a prospective cohort study. Arch Dis Child 2016;101:9–15.
16. American Academy of Pediatrics, Joint Committee on Infant Hearing. Year 2007 position statement: principles and guidelines for early hearing detection and intervention programs. Pediatrics 2007;120:898–921.
17. Harrison M, Roush J, Wallace J. Trends in age of identification and intervention in infants with hearing loss. Ear Hear 2003;24:89–95.
18. Yoshinaga-Itano C, Sedey AL, Coulter DK, et al. Language of early- and later-identified children with hearing loss. Pediatrics 1998;102:1161–71.
19. Mehl AL, Thomson V. The Colorado newborn hearing screening project, 1992-1999: on the threshold of effective population-based universal newborn hearing screening. Pediatrics 2002;109:E7.
20. Vohr BR, Carty LM, Moore PE, et al. The Rhode Island Hearing Assessment Program: experience with statewide hearing screening (1993-1996). J Pediatr 1998;133:353–7.
21. Centers for Disease Control and Prevention (CDC). Identifying infants with hearing loss - United States, 1999-2007. MMWR Morb Mortal Wkly Rep 2010;59:220–3.
22. Campbell K, Mullin G. Otoacoustic emissions. Medscape; 2016.
23. Connolly JL, Carron JD, Roark SD. Universal newborn hearing screening: are we achieving the Joint Committee on Infant Hearing (JCIH) objectives? Laryngoscope 2005;115:232–6.
24. Jakubikova J, Kabatova Z, Pavlovcinova G, et al. Newborn hearing screening and strategy for early detection of hearing loss in infants. Int J Pediatr Otorhinolaryngol 2009;73:607–12.
25. Bray P, Kemp D. An advanced cochlear echo technique suitable for infant screening. Br J Audiol 1987;21:191–204.
26. Lin HC, Shu MT, Lee KS, et al. Comparison of hearing screening programs between one step with transient evoked otoacoustic emissions (TEOAE) and two steps with TEOAE and automated auditory brainstem response. Laryngoscope 2005;115:1957–62.
27. Hahn M, Lamprecht-Dinnesen A, Heinecke A, et al. Hearing screening in healthy newborns: feasibility of different methods with regard to test time. Int J Pediatr Otorhinolaryngol 1999;51:83–9.
28. Benito-Orejas JI, Ramirez B, Morais D, et al. Comparison of two-step transient evoked otoacoustic emissions (TEOAE) and automated auditory brainstem response (AABR) for universal newborn hearing screening programs. Int J Pediatr Otorhinolaryngol 2008;72:1193–201.
29. Hunter MF, Kimm L, Cafarlli Dees D, et al. Feasibility of otoacoustic emission detection followed by ABR as a universal neonatal screening test for hearing impairment. Br J Audiol 1994;28:47–51.
30. Gravel J, Berg A, Bradley M, et al. New York State universal newborn hearing screening demonstration project: effects of screening protocol on inpatient outcome measures. Ear Hear 2000;21:131–40.

31. Levit Y, Himmelfarb M, Dollberg S. Sensitivity of the automated auditory brainstem response in neonatal hearing screening. Pediatrics 2015;136:e641-7.
32. Johnson JL, White KR, Widen JE, et al. A multicenter evaluation of how many infants with permanent hearing loss pass a two-stage otoacoustic emissions/automated auditory brainstem response newborn hearing screening protocol. Pediatrics 2005;116:663-72.
33. Young NM, Reilly BK, Burke L. Limitations of universal newborn hearing screening in early identification of pediatric cochlear implant candidates. Arch Otolaryngol Head Neck Surg 2011;137:230-4.
34. Weichbold V, Nekahm-Heis D, Welzl-Mueller K. Universal newborn hearing screening and postnatal hearing loss. Pediatrics 2006;117:e631-6.
35. Dedhia K, Kitsko D, Sabo D, et al. Children with sensorineural hearing loss after passing the newborn hearing screen. JAMA Otolaryngol Head Neck Surg 2013; 139:119-23.
36. Moore JK, Linthicum FH Jr. The human auditory system: a timeline of development. Int J Audiol 2007;46:460-78.
37. Sleifer P, da Costa SS, Coser PL, et al. Auditory brainstem response in premature and full-term children. Int J Pediatr Otorhinolaryngol 2007;71:1449-56.
38. Hof JR, Stokroos RJ, Wix E, et al. Auditory maturation in premature infants: a potential pitfall for early cochlear implantation. Laryngoscope 2013;123:2013-8.
39. Coenraad S, Goedegebure A, Hoeve LJ. An initial overestimation of sensorineural hearing loss in NICU infants after failure on neonatal hearing screening. Int J Pediatr Otorhinolaryngol 2011;75:159-62.
40. Massinger C, Lippert KL, Keilmann A. [Delay in the development of the auditory pathways. A differential diagnosis in hearing impairment in young infants]. HNO 2004;52:927-34.
41. Talero-Gutierrez C, Carvajalino-Monje I, Samper BS, et al. Delayed auditory pathway maturation in the differential diagnosis of hypoacusis in young children. Int J Pediatr Otorhinolaryngol 2008;72:519-27.
42. Psarommatis I, Florou V, Fragkos M, et al. Reversible auditory brainstem responses screening failures in high risk neonates. Eur Arch Otorhinolaryngol 2011;268:189-96.
43. Strickland J, Needleman A. Auditory electrophysiology. A clinical guide. New York: Thieme Medical Publishers; 2012.
44. Celik O, Eskiizmir G, Uz U. A comparison of thresholds of auditory steady-state response and auditory brainstem response in healthy term babies. J Int Adv Otol 2016;12:277-81.
45. Park AH, Duval M, McVicar S, et al. A diagnostic paradigm including cytomegalovirus testing for idiopathic pediatric sensorineural hearing loss. Laryngoscope 2014;124:2624-9.
46. Liming BJ, Carter J, Cheng A, et al. International Pediatric Otolaryngology Group (IPOG) consensus recommendations: hearing loss in the pediatric patient. Int J Pediatr Otorhinolaryngol 2016;90:251-8.
47. Boone RT, Bower CM, Martin PF. Failed newborn hearing screens as presentation for otitis media with effusion in the newborn population. Int J Pediatr Otorhinolaryngol 2005;69:393-7.
48. Boudewyns A, Declau F, Van den Ende J, et al. Otitis media with effusion: an underestimated cause of hearing loss in infants. Otol Neurotol 2011;32:799-804.
49. Rosenfeld RM, Shin JJ, Schwartz SR, et al. Clinical practice guideline: otitis media with effusion executive summary (update). Otolaryngol Head Neck Surg 2016;154:201-14.

Aspiration and Dysphagia in the Neonatal Patient

Nikhila Raol, MD, MPH[a,b],*, Thomas Schrepfer, MD[a,b], Christopher Hartnick, MD, MS[c]

KEYWORDS

- Dysphagia • Aspiration • Neonate • Feeding difficulty • Failure to thrive
- Aerodigestive

KEY POINTS

- Management of neonatal dysphagia and aspiration should involve a multidisciplinary effort, including neonatologists, otolaryngologists, pulmonologists, gastroenterologists, and speech-language pathologists.
- Flexible fiberoptic laryngoscopy and a formal swallow evaluation in conjunction with the speech pathologist should be undertaken in any neonatal patient with dysphagia.
- Babies born before 34 weeks may have dysphagia owing to a developmental delay.
- Although the otolaryngologist may recommend acid suppression in patients with laryngomalacia, there is a lack of evidence to support use of acid suppression medications in suspected extraesophageal reflux disease.
- Addressing anatomic/structural causes of aspiration are indicated when present; however, the vast majority are nonanatomic.

INTRODUCTION

Dysphagia is defined as difficulty in swallowing and aspiration is defined as the taking of foreign matter into the lungs with the respiratory current. The annual incidence of pediatric swallowing problems in the United States to reported be 0.9%,[1,2] although the incidence of dysphagia is likely much higher in specific populations (neurologic abnormalities, airway anomalies).[3] Unfortunately, data for the prevalence of pediatric swallowing disorders is sparse, especially neonates and infants. Higher rates of aspiration/dysphagia are discovered in children with prematurity, upper aerodigestive tract anomalies, central nervous system malformations, neurodevelopmental delays, and craniofacial syndromes.[4]

The authors have no financial or intellectual relationships to disclose.

[a] Department of Otolaryngology–Head and Neck Surgery, Emory University School of Medicine, 2015 Uppergate Drive, Atlanta, GA 30322, USA; [b] Division of Pediatric Otolaryngology, Children's Healthcare of Atlanta, 2015 Uppergate Drive, Atlanta, GA 30322, USA; [c] Department of Otolaryngology–Head and Neck Surgery, Massachusetts Eye and Ear Infirmary, Harvard Medical School, 243 Charles Street, Boston, MA 02143, USA

* Corresponding author. Emory University School of Medicine, 2015 Uppergate Drive, Atlanta, GA 30322.

E-mail address: npraol@emory.edu

established during the 32nd to 34th weeks of gestational age does not change significantly through 40 weeks. However, the stability of this rhythm increases during that time. The rhythm during this period involves a 1:1 suck to swallow ratio. Differences between males and females have been noted for early activity of oral, lingual, pharyngeal, and laryngeal structures around 24 weeks of age, despite similar physical growth. Females have shown earlier development of complex oral-motor and upper airway skills, with more consistent skills seen in females throughout the second trimester. These differences seem to disappear by the third trimester.[23]

As the neonate reaches full term, the rhythm may advance to a 2:1 to 3:1 suck to swallow ratio. The sucking and swallowing pattern matures from preterm to term infant as evidenced by increased sucking and swallowing rates, longer sucking bursts, and larger volumes per suck.[19] With regard to coordination of the suck–swallow–breathe sequence, during the first week of nipple feeding, minute ventilation, respiratory rate and tidal volumes are expected to decrease sporadically. The majority of swallows are followed by expiration.[24]

The neonatal anatomy of the oral cavity and pharynx at birth are integral to successful early feeding. The mandible is relatively small when compared with the remainder of the skull; therefore, the tongue fills essentially the entire oral cavity, which results in little room for deviation from normal tongue movements. In addition, the fat pads in the cheek narrow the oral cavity. The curvature from the nasopharynx to the oropharynx is a gentle, soft curve, as opposed to the 90° angle in the adult.[22] The larynx is positioned higher (level of the fourth cervical vertebra) in the neonate, just under the tongue, allowing for some protection of the larynx from aspiration.[19] This positioning allows for a smooth backward-forward motion of the tongue to effectively extract milk from the breast or bottle.

It is also critical to understand the complexities of the neural pathways involved in normal swallowing in the neonate. The aerodigestive tract, and the oropharynx in particular, has one of the most abundant and diverse sensory inputs of the entire body.[19] Cranial nerves V, VII, IX, and X provide the majority of afferent input to the brainstem swallowing center from the oropharynx. The nuclei in the brainstem that receive these signals include the rostral nucleus tractus solitarius,[19] but there are also several cortical areas that influence deglutition.[25–27] In addition, the aerodigestive regions have heavy innervation by fibers responding to noxious stimuli, most heavily around the mouth and nose, as well as temperature. The tongue has a high density of mechanosensitive neurons that respond to touch and pressure. Cranial nerves V, VII, IX, X, and XII, as C1 to C3 upper cervical nerves, provide the primary efferent input to the brainstem swallowing centers. The primary laryngeal chemoreflexes that are stimulated when fluid contacts the mucosa of the larynx are startle, rapid swallowing, apnea, laryngeal construction, hypertension, and bradycardia, with rapid swallowing and apnea being most common in neonates. As the neonate matures into an infant and beyond, the likelihood of a cough reflex occurring with fluid contacting the laryngeal surface increases. In addition, rapid swallowing and apnea become less frequent.[28,29]

THE PREMATURE INFANT

Aspiration can be a problem in newborn infants, especially those born prematurely with the inability to coordinate their suck, swallow, and breathing. By 34 weeks of gestational age, however, most infants are able to perform these functions well enough to begin bottle feeding or breastfeeding. The maturation of oral and pharyngeal anatomy and the evolution of the sucking process develop parallel to the development of the brain and nervous system. The correlation between prematurity, complex medical conditions, and feeding disorders in children is well-established.[30,31] Delayed reflexes, hypotonia, and generalized lack of coordination complicate the control of normal swallowing function in developmentally affected children.

Prematurity contributes to a delay in the pharyngeal phase of swallowing and weak suck reflex and is usually complicated by chronic lung disease and neurologic comorbidities, which may be secondary to intraventricular hemorrhage, hypoxia, and neurologic immaturity and development. Given the multifactorial background of dysphagia in preterm infants, they also are more likely to present with poor tone with corresponding laryngomalacia and failure to respond to surgical interventions such as supraglottoplasty, in addition to poor head control, uncoordinated tongue movement, impaired palatal function, poor gag reflex, and laryngopharyngeal hyposensitivity.[32]

Intubation as a newborn can also contribute to aspiration and dysphagia in this population. The presence of an endotracheal tube and the resultant remodeling of the soft palate can lead to velopharyngeal or palatopharyngeal incompetence, nasal reflux, or a defective integration of the suck–swallow mechanism.[4,33] Glottic stenosis, which may result from a prolonged intubation, may lead to aspiration owing to inability to achieve complete glottic closure with swallowing owing to scarring. Conversely, the presence of a tracheostomy tube in a newborn can prevent the normal increase in the subglottic pressure and laryngeal elevation necessary for an effective pharyngeal phase of swallowing.

ANATOMIC ABNORMALITIES CAUSING DYSPHAGIA AND ASPIRATION

Anatomic abnormalities resulting in dysphagia and/or aspiration in the neonate can occur anywhere along the aerodigestive pathway, including the nasal cavity/nasopharynx, oral cavity/oropharynx, and larynx. These abnormalities may include craniofacial anomalies, masses, vascular issues, and a number of other etiologies. Obtaining an accurate history can help with identifying an anatomic reason for dysphagia, including familial/genetic disorders known prenatally, as well as a detailed birth history (ie, prematurity, length of labor, presentation, and trauma during delivery).[34] Here we outline anatomic causes of dysphagia in the neonate.

Nasal Cavity/Nasopharynx

Neonates and infants are considered obligate nasal breathers. Therefore, a decrease in airflow secondary to obstruction of the nose and nasopharynx can lead to significant feeding difficulties owing to interruption of the suck–swallow–breathe mechanism necessary for successful feeding. Nasal obstruction may cause difficulty with feeding in 40% to 50% of these patients.[34] The primary reason for this is the configuration of structures in the oropharynx, with the soft palate nearly contacting the epiglottis, which does not allow for a large amount of space in the oral cavity for airflow. The most common conditions causing nasal obstruction are midface hypoplasia, piriform aperture stenosis, choanal atresia, congenital masses (eg, dacryocystocele, dermoids, encephaloceles, and gliomas), tumors, rhinitis of infancy, and septal deviation.[35] Midface hypoplasia may be seen in syndromic children, such as those with Crouzon and Apert syndromes, as well as children with trisomy 21. Piriform aperture stenosis can be accompanied by holoprosencephaly and a central megaincisor. Choanal atresia may be isolated or part of a syndrome, such as CHARGE syndrome.

Neonates with obstruction at the level of the nasal cavity or nasopharynx typically present with stertor. In the case of bilateral choanal atresia, cyclical cyanosis, with

(GERD) is intimately associated with laryngomalacia and may play a role in the etiology of the disease, including decreased laryngeal sensation secondary to GERD, but a clear causal mechanism has not yet been established.[51,55]

The average age at surgery ranges from 3 to 5 months. Although supraglottoplasty relieves symptoms of upper airway obstruction, it is not without risk (**Box 1**). The most serious complication is supraglottic stenosis and an increased risk of aspiration owing to limited motion and decreased sensation at the level of the supraglottic tissues. Recent studies have suggested that supraglottoplasty does not cause aspiration in patients who did not exhibit aspiration preoperatively. However, it has also been suggested that supraglottoplasty might not relieve aspiration in patients with multiple medical comorbidities.[52] The laryngeal adductor reflex is a sensorimotor reflex that starts with a peripheral afferent laryngeal sensation that travels to the brainstem and stimulates efferent vagal motor responses that cause glottis closure and airway protection during swallowing. The laryngeal adductor reflex is part of one theory behind the correlation between neurologic disorders and postsupraglottoplasty aspiration. It has been demonstrated that the factors that change the peripheral and central reflexes of the laryngeal adductor reflex contribute to the etiology of symptoms and signs of layngomalacia.[55,56]

VFMI, which may be true vocal fold paralysis or just a decrease in full excursion, represents about 10% of congenital laryngeal lesions.[57] Among patients with VFMI, 50% will present with dysphagia.[58] Unilateral VFMI typically presents with hoarseness or a weak cry in conjunction with dysphagia, whereas bilateral VFMI is manifested by respiratory issues, including stridor, apnea, and cyanosis.[59] Causes may include a Chiari malformation, or be iatrogenic owing to thoracic surgery, or idiopathic. Workup includes flexible fiberoptic laryngoscopy, with possible follow-up imaging including computed tomography of the chest or MRI of the brain.[58,60,61] Rates of resolution of VFMI vary in the literature, but what has been demonstrated in a number of studies, irrespective of the etiology, is that dysphagia may improve independent of resolution of VFMI.[58,61] Therefore, even if patients continue to have VFMI, they may learn to overcome the anatomic abnormality and obtain a normal swallow. If surgery is indicated for dysphagia owing to unilateral VFMI, the first-line treatment is injection laryngoplasty, performed under anesthesia. The vocal fold is injected with absorbable material, most commonly carboxymethyl cellulose, which lasts for about 1 to 6 months.

Laryngotracheoesophageal cleft is a rare congenital anomaly consisting of a midline defect along the posterior portion of the larynx and trachea and the anterior portion of the esophagus creating an abnormal communication between the airway at the

---

Box 1
Supraglottoplasty technique

Anesthesiologist administers general anesthesia (keep patient spontaneously breathing if possible).

Insert laryngoscope and apply topical anesthetic.

Perform rigid bronchoscopy (assess for a secondary airway lesions).

Suspend laryngoscope.

Release foreshortened aryepiglottic folds with microlaryngeal scissors.

Trim redundant supraarytenoid tissue with microlaryngeal scissors (care taken not to disturb interarytenoid mucosa).

Obtain hemostasis with oxymetazoline-soaked pledgets.

esophagus. Classification of the cleft depends on length of the communication, ranging from type I (an interarytenoid cleft) to a type IV, which extends below the thoracic inlet.[62] Although flexible fiberoptic laryngoscopy is used to rule out other pathologies, direct laryngoscopy is required for diagnosis of a cleft, particularly for a type I cleft.[63] Often these children are not diagnosed in the neonatal period and may present later with recurrent infections or may already have had a nasogastric tube in place for some time before diagnosis.[64] Depending on the severity of the symptoms, management may include enteral nutrition, thickening of feeds, and/or surgical repair, although this is generally done when the child is older for type I clefts owing to the need for a larger airway to tolerate endoscopic management. In a small group of patients, it is possible that, with feeding therapy alone, dysphagia may resolve, without the need for surgical intervention[65] (Fig. 2).

GASTROESOPHAGEAL REFLUX DISEASE

Gastroesophageal reflux is correlated with intermittent relaxation of the lower esophageal sphincter and resultant ingress of stomach contents into the esophagus.[66,67] When this results in a negative impact on quality of life, it is considered GERD.[68] Symptoms associated with GERD are provided in Table 1.

When testing for GERD, the 2018 North American nor European Societies for Pediatric Gastroenterology, Hepatology, and Nutrition recommend against a number of tests that are routinely used, such as an upper gastrointestinal tract series, ultrasound examination, salivary pepsin, esophageal manometry, and scintigraphy, although these can be used to rule out other etiologies of dysphagia, such as structural abnormalities (upper gastrointestinal series) and esophageal motility disorders (manometry).[69] They also recommend against using pharmacotherapy (proton pump inhibitors) or transpyloric/jejunal feeding trials to attempt to test for GERD in neonates/infants.[69] Recommendations include esophagogastroduodenoscopy with biopsies to assess for complications of GERD, particularly if an underlying mucosal disease is suspected, and multichannel intraluminal impedance testing to correlate persistent worrisome symptoms with acid and nonacid gastroesophageal reflux events and to clarify the role of acid and nonacid reflux in the etiology of esophagitis and other signs and symptoms suggestive of GERD.[69]

The management of GERD should involve a gastroenterologist, and it typically begins with medical therapy. Thickening formula feeds with low or no arsenic rice cereal or using a preprepared thickened formula for full-term infants who are able to tolerate cow's milk protein is an acceptable strategy for otherwise healthy infants with gastroesophageal reflux or GERD.[66,69] A recent Cochrane review demonstrated that formula-fed infants had nearly 2 fewer episodes of regurgitation per day when on thickened feeds; however, data on actually decreasing reflux episodes based on pH probe was of low certainty. In addition, no studies reported the effect on aspiration.[70] If neonates are receiving breastmilk, commercially available thickeners may be used to thicken the milk, but only carob bean thickeners are approved in this population, specifically after 42 weeks of gestation. Xanthum gum-based thickeners are not approved until 1 year of age owing to an association between feed thickening and necrotizing enterocolitis, particularly in preterm infants.[71–73] Modification of feeding is also recommended to avoid overfeeding.[69] When optimal nonpharmacologic treatment fails, a 2- to 4-week trial of extensively hydrolyzed protein-based (or amino acid–based) formula in infants suspected of GERD is recommended before considering any medications for treatment.[69]

NONSURGICAL MANAGEMENT VIA FEEDING MODIFICATION

A number of strategies exist to improve neonatal dysphagia and reduce accompanying sequelae.

- *Pacing*: The goal of pacing is to prevent a stressful scenario related to problems with the suck–swallow–breathe sequence, which may result in desaturations and cause hypoxia.[74,75] Infants who can demonstrate 3 to 5 sucks without taking a breath may be good candidates for pacing. Pacing has been shown to reduce episodes of bradycardia, shorten the duration of stay in the neonatal intensive care unit and promoted efficient sucking and overall more mature feeding behaviors.[76]
- *Modification of feeding position:* The elevated sidelying position has been shown to be effective for feeding, improving oxygen saturation, decreasing heart rate, reducing respiratory rate changes and work of breathing, and generating shorter apneic pauses.[77] Sidelying may also allow for more time to manage flow efficiently, owing to the decrease in the influence of gravity on oral transit time of milk through the aerodigestive tract. This position may allow for more opportunity for improvement of the suck–swallow–breathe sequence.[75]
- *Nipple change*: Slowing down the flow of milk coming from a nipple may improve the efficiency of feeds, thereby improving the suck–swallow–breathe mechanism. Infants fed with slower flow nipples have been found to consume greater volumes, feed faster, and have better sucking efficiency.[78]

SUMMARY

Neonatal dysphagia and aspiration can be difficult to treat. Multiple etiologies can be responsible for feeding and swallowing issues, including prematurity, structural abnormalities, neurologic delay, infectious etiology, and reflux. Identifying the etiology will help to guide management. Most management in the neonatal period is conservative, with medical therapy or supplemental nutrition. In certain etiologies, as in laryngomalacia, surgery may improve dysphagia and allow for return to normal feeding. Multidisciplinary team management, including otolaryngology, neonatologists, speech-language pathologists is necessary to achieve optimal short and long-term outcomes in these patients.

Best Practices

- Evaluation of dysphagia should involve either a videofluoroscopic swallow study or a fiberoptic endoscopic evaluation of the swallow.[63]
- Use nonpharmacotherapy strategies as first-line management of GERD-related dysphagia.[69]
- Surgical intervention should only be undertaken if medical therapy, including nonpharmacologic and pharmacologic treatment, fails, or if there is a concern for airway-related complications or failure to thrive.[53,63,69]

REFERENCES

1. Bhattacharyya N. The prevalence of pediatric voice and swallowing problems in the United States. Laryngoscope 2015;125(3):746–50.
2. Svystun O, Johannsen W, Persad R, et al. Dysphagia in healthy children: characteristics and management of a consecutive cohort at a tertiary centre. Int J Pediatr Otorhinolaryngol 2017;99:54–9.

3. Lefton-Greif MA, McGrath-Morrow SA. Deglutition and respiration: development, coordination, and practical implications. Semin Speech Lang 2007;28(3):166–79.

4. Durvasula VSPB, O'Neill AC, Richter GT. Oropharyngeal dysphagia in children: mechanism, source, and management. Otolaryngol Clin North Am 2014;47(5): 691–720.

5. Jadcherla SR. Advances with neonatal aerodigestive science in the pursuit of safe swallowing in infants: invited review. Dysphagia 2017;32(1):15–26.

6. Adil E, Al Shemari H, Kacprowicz A, et al. Evaluation and management of chronic aspiration in children with normal upper airway anatomy. JAMA Otolaryngol Head Neck Surg 2015;141(11):1006–11.

7. Weir K, McMahon S, Barry L, et al. Clinical signs and symptoms of oropharyngeal aspiration and dysphagia in children. Eur Respir J 2009;33(3):604–11.

8. Suiter DM, Leder SB, Karas DE. The 3-ounce (90-cc) water swallow challenge: a screening test for children with suspected oropharyngeal dysphagia. Otolaryngol Head Neck Surg 2009;140(2):187–90.

9. Bülow M. Videofluoroscopic swallow study: techniques, signs and reports. Nestle Nutr Inst Workshop Ser 2012;72:43–52.

10. Dodrill P, Gosa MM. Pediatric dysphagia: physiology, assessment, and management. Ann Nutr Metab 2015;66(Suppl 5):24–31.

11. Willette S, Molinaro LH, Thompson DM, et al. Fiberoptic examination of swallowing in the breastfeeding infant. Laryngoscope 2016;126(7):1681–6.

12. Bader C-A, Niemann G. Dysphagia in children and young persons. The value of fiberoptic endoscopic evaluation of swallowing. HNO 2008;56(4):397–401 [in German].

13. Boseley ME, Ashland J, Hartnick CJ. The utility of the fiberoptic endoscopic evaluation of swallowing (FEES) in diagnosing and treating children with Type I laryngeal clefts. Int J Pediatr Otorhinolaryngol 2006;70(2):339–43.

14. Sitton M, Arvedson J, Visotcky A, et al. Fiberoptic endoscopic evaluation of swallowing in children: feeding outcomes related to diagnostic groups and endoscopic findings. Int J Pediatr Otorhinolaryngol 2011;75(8):1024–31.

15. Ulualp S, Brown A, Sanghavi R, et al. Assessment of laryngopharyngeal sensation in children with dysphagia. Laryngoscope 2013;123(9):2291–5.

16. Willging JP, Thompson DM. Pediatric FEESST: fiberoptic endoscopic evaluation of swallowing with sensory testing. Curr Gastroenterol Rep 2005;7(3):240–3.

17. Kashou NH, Dar IA, El-Mahdy MA, et al. Brain lesions among orally fed and gastrostomy-fed dysphagic preterm infants: can routine qualitative or volumetric quantitative magnetic resonance imaging predict feeding outcomes? Front Pediatr 2017;5:73.

18. Matsuo K, Palmer JB. Anatomy and physiology of feeding and swallowing: normal and abnormal. Phys Med Rehabil Clin N Am 2008;19(4):691–707, vii.

19. Delaney AL, Arvedson JC. Development of swallowing and feeding: prenatal through first year of life. Dev Disabil Res Rev 2008;14(2):105–17.

20. Derkay CS, Schechter GL. Anatomy and physiology of pediatric swallowing disorders. Otolaryngol Clin North Am 1998;31(3):397–404.

21. Miller CK, Willging JP. Advances in the evaluation and management of pediatric dysphagia. Curr Opin Otolaryngol Head Neck Surg 2003;11(6):442–6.

22. Arvedson JC, Lefton-Greif MA. Anatomy, physiology, and development of feeding. Semin Speech Lang 1996;17(4):261–8.

23. Miller JL, Macedonia C, Sonies BC. Sex differences in prenatal oral-motor function and development. Dev Med Child Neurol 2006;48(6):465–70.

There is a strong genetic component to the development of orofacial clefts. More than 200 genetic syndromes have been associated with cleft lip (CL) and 400 syndromes with cleft palate (CP).[6] Frequently discussed genetic syndromes with genes associated with orofacial clefts include CHARGE syndrome (CHD7), velocardiofacial syndrome (TBX1, COMT), and Apert syndrome (FGFR2).[7] The genetic component to orofacial clefting is also demonstrated in the increased recurrence rate among affected families. Each child of an affected parent with a cleft has a 3% risk of having an orofacial cleft. If one sibling is affected, the risk of a cleft in subsequent children is 5%. If both a sibling and parent are affected, there is a 14% risk of cleft formation in subsequent children.[8]

Multiple environmental factors have also been linked with CLP. Risk factors include smoking, pregestational and gestational diabetes, alcohol abuse, and certain anticonvulsants.[9–11] Specific nutritional deficiencies that may contribute to the risk of clefting include inadequate folate and vitamins B_6 and B_{12}.[3,12] Providing further evidence for the role of maternal nutrition in lip and palate development, a systematic review found that maternal multivitamin use resulted in a 25% decrease in the odds of a child being born with a cleft.[13]

Embryology of Cleft Lip and Palate

Lip embryologic development begins at gestational week 4 with the appearance of the paired maxillary prominences and the unpaired frontonasal prominence (**Fig. 1**A–D). In week 5, the medial and lateral nasal processes develop from the invagination of the nasal placodes. The paired maxillary prominences extend medially in weeks 6 to 7 and meet the nasal processes to form the upper lip.

The primary palate develops from the fusion of the paired medial nasal prominences in weeks 6 to 7 (**Fig. 1**E–H). This fusion forms the intermaxillary segment, which will contain the central 4 incisors and hard palate anterior to the incisive foramen. At this time, palatine processes or shelves also extend medially from the paired maxillary

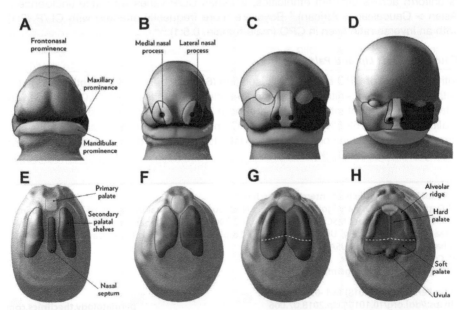

Fig. 1. (*A–D*) Upper lip development sequence. (*E–H*) Soft and hard palate development (*Illustration by Emma Vought*).

prominences. Fusion of the palatal shelves to form the secondary palate begins in week 9 (fusion begins anteriorly at the incisive foramen and extends posteriorly to the uvula).

Classification of Cleft Lip and Palate

CLs can be classified as microform, incomplete, or complete. A microform CL describes a notch or groove in the soft tissues of the lip (**Fig. 2**A). All of the lip tissues are present, but there is a notch at the vermilion-cutaneous junction. In contrast, incomplete CLs involve dehiscence of the orbicularis oris and can be variable in their involvement of the skin (**Fig. 2**B). A Simonart band refers to a thin band of soft tissue that spans the superior aspect of an incomplete CL at the nasal sill. Complete CLs extend through the length of the lip and into the nasal sill, leading to abnormal insertion of the orbicularis oris onto the ala and columella (**Fig. 2**C). In addition, in bilateral CL

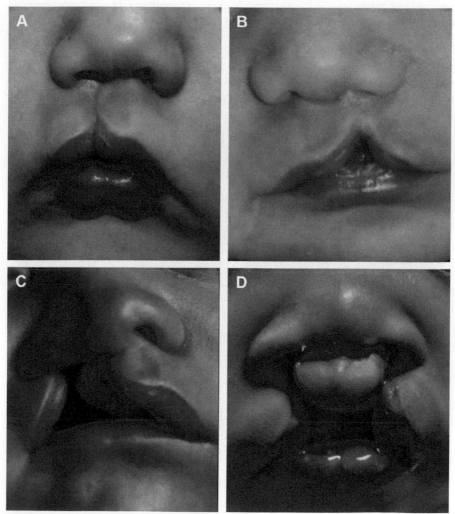

Fig. 2. (*A*) Microform right CL. (*B*) Incomplete left CL. (*C*) Complete right CL. (*D*) Bilateral complete CL.

there is anterior displacement of the intermaxillary segment with absence of the orbicularis oris within the intermaxillary segment (**Fig. 2**D).

CPs can likewise be classified by the extent of their anatomic involvement. Submucous CPs are characterized by an underlying dehiscence of the palatal musculature, whereas the overlying mucosa is intact. Because they do not have an associated mucosal defect, detection of submucous CPs can be challenging. Physical examination findings associated with a submucous CP include midline notching of the hard palate, bifid uvula, and a zona pellucida (blue line in the midline of the soft palate representing the lack of musculature and increased transparency). A cleft of the secondary palate involves a defect extending posteriorly from the incisive foramen through the soft palate to the uvula. In contrast, a cleft of the primary palate involves the palate anterior to the incisive foramen extending to the alveolar arch. A complete CP involves both the primary and secondary palates. Examples of the different types of CP are shown in **Fig. 3**. Note that primary and secondary palate describe the palate by its embryologic origins. In contrast, the terms hard and soft palate refer to the anatomic findings represented by the anterior bony palate and the posterior soft tissue/musculature palate, respectively.

Prenatal Diagnosis of Cleft Lip and Palate

Birthing and raising a child with orofacial clefting can be a source of psychological distress for mothers and families.[14,15] Antenatal diagnosis of an orofacial cleft allows for prenatal counseling and can assist families in being prepared for the care of their

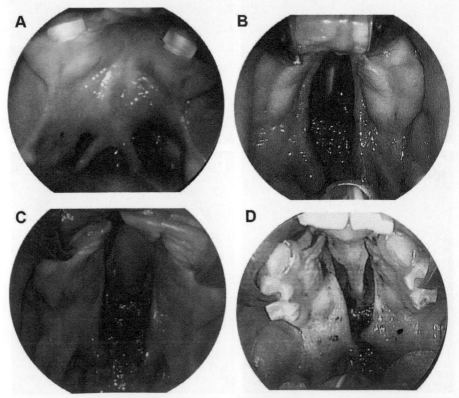

Fig. 3. (*A*) Submucous CP. (*B*) Incomplete CP. (*C*) Unilateral complete CP. (*D*) Bilateral complete CP.

future child.[16,17] Prenatal diagnosis also allows families to meet the craniofacial team members before birth and can help facilitate the recommended early postpartum evaluation of affected infants.

In the United States, anatomic ultrasonography studies are frequently obtained between 18 and 20 weeks' gestation. The accuracy of two-dimensional (2D) ultrasonography in detecting an orofacial cleft among low-risk patients is variable, with detection rates of 0% to 70% reported in a systematic review.[18] Infants with CPO are less likely to be detected than those with CL/P.[18] The prenatal ultrasonography detection rate is likely dependent on multiple factors, including sonographer experience, gestational age, and whether the laboratory routinely performs imaging of the face. Compared with 2D studies, three-dimensional (3D) ultrasonography has an increased diagnostic accuracy in general, and has shown an ability to detect a CP when a CL has been previously detected on 2D ultrasonography (up to 100% sensitivity).[18,19]

Early Multidisciplinary Evaluation

The American Cleft Palate-Craniofacial Association emphasizes the importance of multidisciplinary treatment of these patients within the first few days of life.[20] Given the frequency of concomitant abnormalities, an early dysmorphology evaluation is essential. If there are additional abnormalities, a comprehensive genetics evaluation should be considered. Once an infant is connected to a craniofacial team, a coordinator can also assist families in planning their follow-up care after discharge. Frequently, patients with CLP require the care of multiple medical specialties (**Table 1**) and should be followed in a multidisciplinary clinic until early adulthood.

Feeding Evaluation

Early feeding difficulties are common among infants with CLP. Issues with nutritional intake can stem from difficulty creating a seal in patients with CL, or an inability to generate the negative pressure or suction to feed in patients with CP.[21] Alterations in

Table 1 Basic cleft care		
Age	**Medical Treatments**	**Surgery**
Prenatal to birth	• Genetic counseling • SLP consultation for feeding	—
0–5 mo	• SLP for feeding and growth • Monitor hearing • NAM (if indicated)	• CL repair • Ear tubes (if COM)
9–12 mo	—	• Palatoplasty • Ear tubes (if COM)
1–4 y	• Introduction to pediatric dentist • Assess language development	—
4–6 y	• Assess for VPD	• Corrective speech surgery • Lip revision if needed • Minor nasal surgery if needed
6–12 y	• Orthodontics • Assess school/psychosocial adjustment	• Alveolar bone grafting
12–21 y	• Orthodontics	• Orthognathic surgery • Definitive rhinoplasty

Abbreviations: COM, chronic otitis media; NAM, nasoalveolar molding; SLP, speech-language pathology; VPD, velopharyngeal dysfunction.

these normal feeding patterns place children with orofacial clefts at increased risk for poor weight gain and dehydration.[22,23] Mothers with infants struggling with feeding are also susceptible to depression, which can further complicate their children's care.[23]

Given the prevalence of feeding difficulties in the cleft population, affected newborns should be seen by a speech-language pathologist, who can perform an evaluation and provide counseling. Typically, patients with CL are able to breastfeed, whereas those with a CP are usually unsuccessful. The authors encourage families of children with CPs to bottle feed for nutrition, but then they may breastfeed briefly as desired for mother and infant bonding. There are multiple cleft-specific bottles, including the Haberman Feeder, Pigeon Feeder, Mead Johnson Cleft Lip/Palate Nurser, and the Dr. Brown's Specialty Feeding System. These bottles can be broadly classified into 2 types: assisted-delivery (squeeze) versus rigid bottles. Assisted-delivery bottles (Haberman and Mead Johnson) are compressible and allow parents to squeeze the reservoir and increase the milk/formula flow. In contrast, rigid bottles (Pigeon and Dr. Brown's) allow the infant to release the flow of milk by compressing the specialized nipple. A Cochrane Review evaluating squeezable versus rigid bottle use among patients with clefts found no evidence for a difference in growth outcome based on bottle choice.[24] As a result, families should be counseled to use whichever bottle works best for their individual child.

Early Cleft Interventions

Both lip taping and nasoalveolar molding (NAM) are frequently used during the neonatal period in an attempt to reduce the severity of a cleft deformity. Suggested benefits of these interventions include decreased cleft width, improved nasal symmetry, and improved psychological outcomes for caregivers.[25–28] However, controversy remains regarding the efficacy of individual techniques and there is a wide variation in clinical practice patterns.[29,30]

Preoperative lip taping is commonly used in children with CLs during the neonatal period.[28,31] At our institution we routinely perform lip taping in infants with complete CL. Beginning within 1 week of life, the tape is applied across the cleft while squeezing the lip together (**Fig. 4**). Before discharge, families are instructed on how to apply the tape daily and are scheduled for follow-up in the cleft surgeon's clinic. The most common complication of lip taping is skin irritation. If this is encountered, a dressing can be placed to protect the skin before taping.

NAM is frequently used at our institution in patients with wide unilateral or bilateral CL/P. Some proposed benefits of NAM include improved nasal symmetry in unilateral CL deformities, increasing columellar length in bilateral CL deformities, and improved alignment of the alveolar arches.[26,32–35] However, NAM involves a commitment from the family. An early family meeting should review the time commitment and the need for frequent initial clinic visits for adjustments to the prosthetic. Once the family and craniofacial team (cleft surgeon, prosthodontist) agree to proceed with NAM, a maxillary impression must be taken (typically within the first weeks of life) (**Fig. 5**). The impression can be taken in the clinic or operating room depending on the comfort level of the prosthodontist. The family is then seen by the prosthodontist within a week for the initial fitting. The parents are instructed on how to apply the NAM and it is worn 24 hours a day. Children are seen every 1 to 2 weeks in clinic for up to 6 months to assess prosthetic fit and treatment effects. The most common reported complications of NAM include skin irritation, poor compliance, and failure of the device to remain in place.[36] The last 2 complications emphasize the importance of patient and family selection because a family not committed to the process is unlikely to have satisfactory compliance or outcome. If NAM is not a possibility, the family is encouraged to use lip taping.

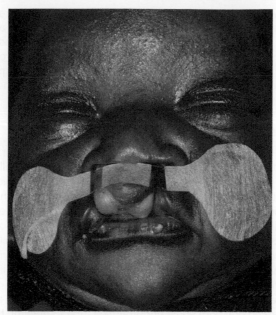

Fig. 4. Patient with bilateral CLP with lip taping in place to apply pressure to reposition the intermaxillary segment posteriorly.

SURGICAL MANAGEMENT
Cleft Lip Preoperative Planning

Lip adhesion may be used for patients with a wide unilateral or bilateral CL who are unable to complete either lip taping or NAM. This surgery is typically performed at age 1 month in preparation for a second-stage lip repair.

Definitive lip repair commonly occurs at age 3 months (or 10 weeks) to avoid airway difficulty associated with obligate nasal breathing in early infancy and postanesthetic apnea. Other factors involved in timing of surgery include weight (ideally ≥4.5 kg [10lb]) and hemoglobin level (ideally 10 g/dL), known as the rule of 10s and first described by Wilhelmsen and Musgrave.[37,38] Adequate completion of NAM or taping

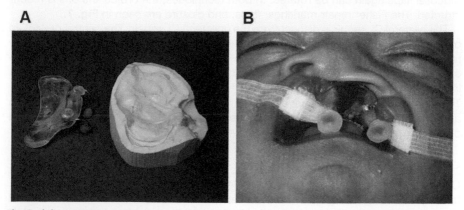

Fig. 5. (A) NAM impression and prosthesis. (B) Patient with unilateral CLP with NAM in place. (Courtesy of Betsy K. Davis, DMD, Medical University of South Carolina, Charleston, SC.)

may defer surgery. Caregivers should be counseled preoperatively regarding risks of surgery to include dehiscence, hypertrophic scar, poor cosmesis, and presence of nasolabial fistula. Technique of feeding (ie, bottle vs syringe) and need for hospitalization after surgery should be discussed as well. Wound care after surgery may involve gentle cleaning and application of ointment unless surgical glue is applied. If permanent cutaneous sutures are used, a second procedure to remove the sutures will be necessary.

Surgical Procedure

The investigators use either the Millard or Fisher technique for repair of the unilateral CL and the Millard technique for repair of the bilateral CL.[39–41] The Millard technique is based on rotation-advancement principles, whereas the Fisher technique is described as an anatomic subunit approach. Other rotation-advancement techniques by Mohler[42] and Noordhoff[43] are also frequently used by surgeons in the United States. The specific surgical technique is commonly used by a surgeon for repair of both incomplete and complete CL.[30] The goals of both unilateral and bilateral CL repair include (1) oral competence via a complete orbicularis oris, (2) symmetry, and (3) cosmesis. A tip rhinoplasty may be performed during this surgery to improve the contour, shape, position, and width of the affected ala and nasal tip.

Lip repair or cheiloplasty is performed under general endotracheal anesthesia, typically with the use of an oral right angle endotracheal tube to position the endotracheal tube inferiorly and out of the surgical field. Local anesthesia is used per surgeon preference. For the Millard repair, critical markings include the high and low points of the Cupid's bow, columellar base, alar bases, and choice of the appropriate high point of Cupid's bow on the lateral lip of the cleft side.[41] The basic principle of the Millard repair is to rotate the noncleft side inferiorly and advance the lateral lip of the cleft side. The C flap originates from the medial non-CL and may be incorporated into the columella for lengthening or the nasal sill. Mucosal M and L flaps can be rotated to bridge the alveolus and minimize the resulting fistula. The aforementioned markings, flaps, and closure for the Millard repair are shown in **Fig. 6**. For the Fisher repair, 25 critical markings are used.[39] A triangle is incorporated into the cutaneous skin at the cleft side philtral column from the lateral lip using predetermined calculations related to the philtral column height of the cleft and noncleft sides. The Rose-Thompson effect adds 1 mm of lengthening. A second triangle is incorporated from the lateral lip vermilion as well. Mucosal flaps again can be rotated. In both techniques, the orbicularis oris is reconstructed. The Fisher repair markings, flaps, and closure are seen in **Fig. 7**.

The bilateral CL repair is distinct from the unilateral CL repair. The central prolabium of the bilateral cleft defect does not contain orbicularis oris muscle and thus surgery requires additional mobilization of the muscle across the premaxilla for adequate muscle reapproximation. The columella is also typically deficient in the bilateral CL. Markings for the bilateral CL repair are similar to those for the unilateral CL repair by Millard. The distinct difference is the advancement of the lateral lip vermilion to the midline to approximate the central low point of Cupid's bow inferiorly. Markings, flaps, and closure for the bilateral CL repair are shown in **Fig. 8**.

Complications

Complications of unilateral CL repair include deficient vermilion or a whistle deformity, under-rotation of the high point on the cleft side, muscular dehiscence, and nasal asymmetry. Secondary surgery for the lip is typically considered at approximately age 5 years or older.

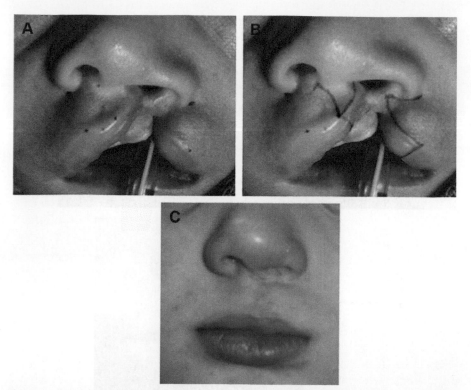

Fig. 6. Unilateral CL repair with Millard technique. (*A*) Surgical markings. (*B*) Flaps. (*C*) Postoperative result.

Cleft Palate Preoperative Planning

Palatoplasty typically occurs between 9 and 12 months of age. Dorf and Curtin[44] showed significantly improved speech outcomes if soft palate repair occurred before age 12 months. Two-stage palate repair with early soft palate closure and delayed hard palate closure is performed as well. Considerations for timing of surgery include the surgery's impact on the oropharyngeal airway and potential disruption of maxillary growth caused by hard palate dissection.

Risks of surgery should be discussed with caregivers before surgery to include fistula, velopharyngeal dysfunction (VPD), maxillary growth disturbance, and sleep-disordered breathing.[45] Short-term complications include hemorrhage, infection, tongue edema, and respiratory difficulty. Need for postoperative hospitalization and feeding plan (ie, bottle vs open-flow cup) should also be included in the preoperative discussion. The goals of palatoplasty include restoration of an intact levator palatini with palatal lengthening; ideally, surgery should have a low incidence of palatal fistula, VPD, and maxillary growth disturbance.

Surgical Procedure

Surgical technique may be selected based on type of palatal involvement (ie, only soft palate vs incomplete secondary palate vs complete secondary palate) and width of the cleft between palatal shelves. The hard palate is repaired with axial mucoperiosteal flaps based on the greater palatine arteries.[46] Vomer flaps may be included to

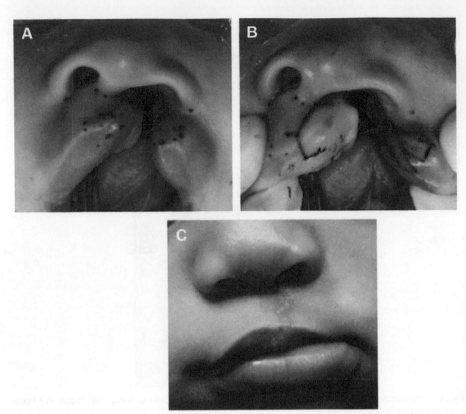

Fig. 7. Unilateral CL repair with Fisher technique. (*A*) Surgical markings. (*B*) Flaps. (*C*) Postoperative result.

aid in nasal closure. Relaxing incisions at the lateral aspect of the hard palate are used for mobility; the lateral donor sites heal by secondary intention with remucosalization. The soft palate is repaired with repositioning of the levator muscle into an intact sling by varying techniques, including a straight-line repair, intravelar veloplasty, or double opposing Z-plasty.[46–48] Regardless of technique, a multilayer closure is used to minimize risk of fistula formation. Markings, flaps, and closure of CPs are shown in **Fig. 9**.

Complications

Long-term complications of palatoplasty include palatal fistula, obstructive sleep apnea (OSA), and VPD. Fistula formation may lead to nasal regurgitation of oral intake and hypernasality. Techniques for palatal fistula closure are beyond the scope of this article but can be complex. OSA has a higher incidence in patients with clefting; screening for symptoms of sleep-disordered breathing should regularly occur in this patient population.[49] A polysomnogram is recommended before additional surgical intervention given their high-risk status.[50] VPD is discussed further later in this article.

COMMON COMORBIDITIES
Hearing and Middle Ear Disease

After the introduction of the newborn hearing screen (NBHS) in the United States, more than 95% of newborn infants are screened in the perinatal period for hearing

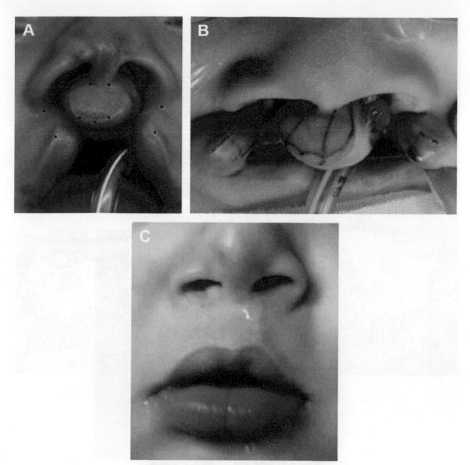

Fig. 8. Bilateral CL repair. (*A*) Surgical markings. (*B*) Flaps. A natal tooth is shown in the premaxilla. (*C*) Postoperative result.

loss with the goal of early identification and intervention.[51] Infants with a cleft anomaly, especially CP, are at higher risk for referring the NBHS.[52] Although this finding is often attributed to middle ear effusion because of the high prevalence of middle ear disease in children with CP, the incidences of sensorineural hearing loss, conductive hearing loss (CHL), and mixed hearing loss are also higher in children with clefting.[52–54]

Eustachian tube dysfunction (ETD), including chronic middle ear effusion, is found in at least 95% of patients with a cleft, specifically CP. The cause of chronic middle ear disease is attributed to anatomic disruption of the tensor veli palatini and change in eustachian tube compliance.[55,56] CHL is found in most patients with a CP because of middle ear findings.[57] Interventions to improve hearing include placement of tympanostomy tubes, palatoplasty, and/or hearing amplification.[58,59] Most children with a CP have improvement in ETD, middle ear disorders, and also hearing by approximately age 6 years.[60] However, there remains a significantly increased incidence of hearing loss in patients with a CP in subsequent years.[58,61]

Tympanostomy tube placement may occur in coordination with CLP repair or additional surgeries to minimize anesthesia exposure, as seen in **Table 1**. Patients with a CP undergo a mean of 3 to 4 tympanostomy tube placement procedures before

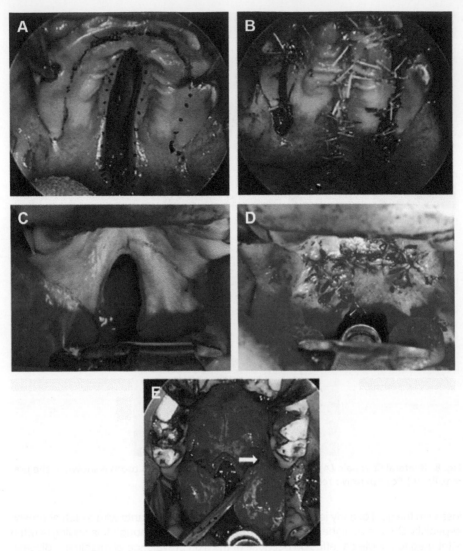

Fig. 9. Palate repair. (*A*) Straight line palatoplasty surgical markings. (*B*) Straight line pala- toplasty outcome. (*C*) Double opposing Z-plasty surgical markings. (*D*) Double opposing Z-plasty outcome. (*E*) Mucoperiosteal flaps for hard palate closure; white arrow indicates greater palatine artery vascular pedicle.

improvement in chronic middle ear disease.[53] A greater risk of persistent CHL exists among patients with multiple sets of tympanostomy tubes or cholesteatoma.[53,62] Because of a higher incidence of cholesteatoma in at-risk patients with persistent middle ear dysfunction, otologic follow-up into adulthood is recommended.[53]

Velopharyngeal Dysfunction

VPD is inadequate closure of the velopharynx during speech such that air escape oc- curs through the nose during oral consonant production with hypernasal resonance. Nasal phonemes (/m/,/n/,/ng/) occur naturally with nasal resonance and an open velopharynx; all other phonemes require closure of the velopharyngeal complex such that the palate elevates to contact the posterior pharyngeal wall. VPD can be subcategorized as velopharyngeal mislearning (often caused by articulation errors and incorrect placement or closure), velopharyngeal incompetency (functional deficit), or velopharyngeal insufficiency (structural or anatomic deficit).

VPD occurs in an estimated 20% of patients who previously underwent CP repair, although the incidence of VPD varies widely in the literature.[63] Risk factors for VPD include history of CP, especially with delayed CP repair; submucous CP; change in velopharyngeal anatomy (ie, adenoidectomy or maxillary advancement); syndromic association including trisomy 21, 22q11.2 deletion syndrome, Kabuki syndrome; or acquired pharyngeal dysfunction or hypotonia (ie, stroke, head injury, head and neck cancer with anatomic defect, or radiation exposure). The double opposing Z-plasty or Furlow palatoplasty has been shown to have improved speech outcomes such that need for a secondary operation because of VPD is lower in children who underwent Furlow repair compared with straight-line closure.[64]

Screening for VPD should begin at an early age (approximately 18 months) for children with a CP and continue at regular intervals into early adulthood. A skilled speech-language pathologist performs a perceptual assessment and/or objective testing using nasometry or pressure flow testing. Adequate speech assessment requires patient maturity and may not be thorough until age 4 or 5 years. Additional testing for VPD includes nasal endoscopy and/or video fluoroscopy to better determine the pattern of velopharyngeal closure and assist with surgical planning. Surgery may ideally be tailored to closure pattern: coronal, sagittal, circular, or circular with Passavant ridge.

Speech therapy may be the primary treatment or an adjunctive treatment preoperatively and/or postoperatively. Therapy is the treatment of choice for velopharyngeal mislearning. Often speech therapy is needed to correct compensatory articulation errors even when surgery is required for an anatomic or structural deficit.

Patients who are not surgical candidates because of airway concerns, prior failed surgeries, existing comorbidities, position of internal carotid arteries, and so forth may be candidates for a prosthesis. A partnership between speech-language pathology and maxillofacial prosthodontics is advantageous to fashion an obturator or palatal lift for these patients.[65] Adequate maxillary dentition is important for prosthesis use.

Surgical interventions for VPD are ideally tailored to closure pattern based on endoscopy or fluoroscopy findings and include (1) posterior pharyngeal wall augmentation, (2) palatal lengthening, and/or (3) alteration of the velopharynx. Small central gaps may be improved with injection pharyngoplasty; various materials have been described for this procedure.[66] If there is evidence of levator muscular dehiscence, double opposing Z-plasty can be used to reorient the levator sling, positioning it posteriorly with added palatal length.[67] This secondary palatal technique may also be used in combination with the sphincter pharyngoplasty. The velopharynx may be altered via (1) sphincter pharyngoplasty or (2) posterior pharyngeal flap. Ideal candidates for sphincter pharyngoplasty are patients with coronal closure patterns and limited lateral pharyngeal wall motion. A sphincter is created via elevation of bilateral superiorly based myomucosal flaps that are inset to the central posterior pharyngeal wall at the level of velar closure.[68] Posterior pharyngeal flap surgery involves elevation of a central superiorly based myomucosal flap that is inset into a submucosal pocket of the soft palate or the central soft palate. A pharyngeal flap should be considered in patients with good lateral pharyngeal wall movement and sagittal or circular closure patterns.[69] Success rates between sphincter pharyngoplasty and pharyngeal flap are similar.[69,70] Complications after secondary speech surgery include persistent

24. Bessell A, Hooper L, Shaw WC, et al. Feeding interventions for growth and development in infants with cleft lip, cleft palate or cleft lip and palate. Cochrane Database Syst Rev 2011;(2):CD003315.

25. Sischo L, Clouston SA, Phillips C, et al. Caregiver responses to early cleft palate care: a mixed method approach. Health Psychol 2016;35(5):474–82.

26. van der Heijden P, Dijkstra PU, Stellingsma C, et al. Limited evidence for the effect of presurgical nasoalveolar molding in unilateral cleft on nasal symmetry: a call for unified research. Plast Reconstr Surg 2013;131(1):62e–71e.

27. Sabarinath VP, Thombare P, Hazarey PV, et al. Changes in maxillary alveolar morphology with nasoalveolar molding. J Clin Pediatr Dent 2010;35(2):207–12.

28. Pool R. Tissue mobilization with preoperative lip taping. Operat Tech Plast Reconstr Surg 1995;2(3):155–8.

29. Rodman RE, Tatum S. Controversies in the management of patients with cleft lip and palate. Facial Plast Surg Clin North Am 2016;24(3):255–64.

30. Sitzman TJ, Girotto JA, Marcus JR. Current surgical practices in cleft care: unilateral cleft lip repair. Plast Reconstr Surg 2008;121(5):261e–70e.

31. Pool R, Farnworth TK. Preoperative lip taping in the cleft lip. Ann Plast Surg 1994; 32(3):243–9.

32. Bennun RD, Perandones C, Sepliarsky VA, et al. Nonsurgical correction of nasal deformity in unilateral complete cleft lip: a 6-year follow-up. Plast Reconstr Surg 1999;104(3):616–30.

33. Barillas I, Dec W, Warren SM, et al. Nasoalveolar molding improves long-term nasal symmetry in complete unilateral cleft lip-cleft palate patients. Plast Reconstr Surg 2009;123(3):1002–6.

34. Broder HL, Flores RL, Clouston S, et al. Surgeon's and caregivers' appraisals of primary cleft lip treatment with and without nasoalveolar molding: a prospective multicenter pilot study. Plast Reconstr Surg 2016;137(3):938–45.

35. Lee CT, Garfinkle JS, Warren SM, et al. Nasoalveolar molding improves appearance of children with bilateral cleft lip-cleft palate. Plast Reconstr Surg 2008; 122(4):1131–7.

36. Levy-Bercowski D, Abreu A, DeLeon E, et al. Complications and solutions in presurgical nasoalveolar molding therapy. Cleft Palate Craniofac J 2009;46(5): 521–8.

37. Wilhelmsen HR, Musgrave RH. Complications of cleft lip surgery. Cleft Palate J 1966;3:223–31.

38. Chow I, Purnell CA, Hanwright PJ, et al. Evaluating the rule of 10s in cleft lip repair: do data support dogma? Plast Reconstr Surg 2016;138(3):670–9.

39. Fisher DM. Unilateral cleft lip repair: an anatomical subunit approximation technique. Plast Reconstr Surg 2005;116(1):61–71.

40. Millard DR Jr. Closure of bilateral cleft lip and elongation of columella by two operations in infancy. Plast Reconstr Surg 1971;47(4):324–31.

41. Millard D, editor. Cleft craft: the evolution of its surgery. Boston: Little; 1976. p. 165–73.

42. Mohler LR. Unilateral cleft lip repair. Plast Reconstr Surg 1987;80(4):511–7.

43. Noordhoff MS. Reconstruction of vermilion in unilateral and bilateral cleft lips. Plast Reconstr Surg 1984;73(1):52–61.

44. Dorf DS, Curtin JW. Early cleft palate repair and speech outcome. Plast Reconstr Surg 1982;70(1):74–81.

45. Chepla KJ, Gosain AK. Evidence-based medicine: cleft palate. Plast Reconstr Surg 2013;132(6):1644–8.

46. Bardach J, Salyer KE. Cleft palate repair. Surgical techniques in cleft lip and palate. St. Louis (MO): Mosby; 1991. p. 224–73.
47. Furlow LT Jr. Cleft palate repair by double opposing Z-plasty. Plast Reconstr Surg 1986;78(6):724–38.
48. Cutting CB, Rosenbaum J, Rovati L. The technique of muscle repair in the cleft soft palate. Operat Tech Plast Reconstr Surg 1995;2:215–22.
49. Muntz H, Wilson M, Park A, et al. Sleep disordered breathing and obstructive sleep apnea in the cleft population. Laryngoscope 2008;118(2):348–53.
50. Marcus CL, Brooks LJ, Draper KA, et al. Diagnosis and management of childhood obstructive sleep apnea syndrome. Pediatrics 2012;130(3): e714–55.
51. Hayes D. State programs for universal newborn hearing screening. Pediatr Clin North Am 1999;46(1):89–94.
52. Chen JL, Messner AH, Curtin G. Newborn hearing screening in infants with cleft palates. Otol Neurotol 2008;29(6):812–5.
53. Goudy S, Lott D, Canady J, et al. Conductive hearing loss and otopathology in cleft palate patients. Otolaryngol Head Neck Surg 2006;134(6):946–8.
54. Anteunis LJ, Brienesse P, Schrander JJ. Otoacoustic emissions in screening cleft lip and/or palate children for hearing loss–a feasibility study. Int J Pediatr Otorhinolaryngol 1998;44(3):259–66.
55. Doyle WJ, Cantekin EI, Bluestone CD. Eustachian tube function in cleft palate children. Ann Otol Rhinol Laryngol Suppl 1980;89(3 Pt 2):34–40.
56. Takahashi H, Honjo I, Fujita A. Eustachian tube compliance in cleft palate–a preliminary study. Laryngoscope 1994;104(1 Pt 1):83–6.
57. Fria TJ, Paradise JL, Sabo DL, et al. Conductive hearing loss in infants and young children with cleft palate. J Pediatr 1987;111(1):84–7.
58. Gould HJ. Hearing loss and cleft palate: the perspective of time. Cleft Palate J 1990;27(1):36–9.
59. Bellis ME, Passy V. Long-term hearing effects in cleft palate patients. Ear Nose Throat J 1987;66(10):409–14.
60. Smith TL, DiRuggiero DC, Jones KR. Recovery of eustachian tube function and hearing outcome in patients with cleft palate. Otolaryngol Head Neck Surg 1994;111(4):423–9.
61. Moller P. Long-term otologic features of cleft palate patients. Arch Otolaryngol 1975;101(10):605–7.
62. Sheahan P, Miller I, Sheahan JN, et al. Incidence and outcome of middle ear disease in cleft lip and/or cleft palate. Int J Pediatr Otorhinolaryngol 2003;67(7): 785–93.
63. Witt PD, D'Antonio LL. Velopharyngeal insufficiency and secondary palatal management. A new look at an old problem. Clin Plast Surg 1993;20(4): 707–21.
64. Timbang MR, Gharb BB, Rampazzo A, et al. A systematic review comparing Furlow double-opposing Z-plasty and straight-line intravelar veloplasty methods of cleft palate repair. Plast Reconstr Surg 2014;134(5):1014–22.
65. Aboloyoun AI, Ghorab S, Farooq MU. Palatal lifting prosthesis and velopharyngeal insufficiency: preliminary report. Acta Med Acad 2013;42(1):55–60.
66. Perez CF, Brigger MT. Posterior pharyngeal wall augmentation. Adv Otorhinolaryngol 2015;76:74–80.
67. Sie KC, Tampakopoulou DA, Sorom J, et al. Results with Furlow palatoplasty in management of velopharyngeal insufficiency. Plast Reconstr Surg 2001;108(1): 17–25 [discussion: 26–9].

Malformations refer to deficient growth of structures resulting from disrupted embryogenesis. Microtia is an example of a malformation and can occur in isolation or as a component of a more encompassing syndrome.

Microtia refers to incomplete embryonic development of the components of the external ear.

Ear deformities associated with restricted growth will be discussed briefly in order to help differentiate from microtia. Recognition of microtia can help the neonatal provider counsel families and search for associated anomalies that can potentially provide insight into an overarching diagnosis.

Children with microtia may have other congenital facial anomalies due to abnormal development or growth of associated embryologic structures. Facial anomalies that are mild or asymptomatic do not require intervention although many will require surgery for functional as well as cosmetic purposes.

The cause of facial anomalies is multifactorial in many cases without a definite cause. However, there is a heavy genetic component to many of these findings. Consultation with a geneticist is indicated to help identify other anatomic and developmental abnormalities that may coexist. Environmental prenatal factors including teratogens and prenatal vitamin use may also play a part in these conditions.

Microtia is a common congenital facial anomaly and in some cases is associated with an underlying syndrome with characteristic facial anomalies. In addition to the cause and management of microtia, this article also discusses the description and management of associated facial anomalies: mandibular and maxillary hypoplasia, temporomandibular joint dysplasia, orbital deformity, and macrostomia.

EAR DEFORMITIES (NONMICROTIA EAR ANOMALIES)

With rare exceptions, such as branchio-oto-renal syndrome (BOR), ear deformities are not usually associated with other physical anomalies or systemic disease. These deformities include underdevelopment of the helix, the lobule, or any other portion of the pinna. Common examples include cup ear, lop ear, Stahl ear, and cryptotia (**Fig. 1**).

BOR is characterized by branchial cleft anomalies and abnormal renal structure and function in addition to bilateral ear anomalies. The incidence of BOR is 1:40,000 births.[1,2] Associated ear anomalies include preauricular pits (80%) or accessory skin/cartilage (ear tags), in addition to the distorted shape of the ears. Renal anomalies and branchial cleft cysts are also common features of BOR. Microtia, however, is not commonly associated with BOR.

EAR MALFORMATIONS

Microtia is the major type of ear malformation. Typically, microtia is graded based on severity as depicted in **Fig. 2**.

EMBRYOLOGY OF MICROTIA

The ear canal begins development during the fifth week of gestation, with the external ear, or auricle, differentiating during the seventh week. The auricle is a derivative of the first and second branchial arches. The first arch gives rise to the first 3 hillocks of His, which form the tragus, helix, and concha cymba. The second branchial arch gives rise to the hillocks 4 to 6, which form the cavum concha, antihelix, and antitragus (**Fig. 3**).

The mandible, maxilla, and associated neuromuscular structures are also derived from the first and second branchial arches. Thus, an early insult to these arches can have wide-reaching alterations in facial development resulting in a variety of

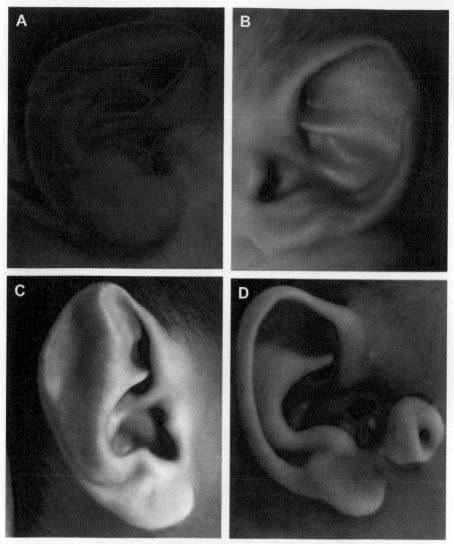

Fig. 1. (*A*) Lop ear, (*B*) flattened scapha, (*C*) Stahl ear, (*D*) duplicated auricle with rudimentary duplicate external auditory canal.

craniofacial syndromes. These anomalies and syndromes associated with microtia will be discussed in more detail later in this article.

EPIDEMIOLOGY OF MICROTIA

The incidence of microtia is estimated to be 1:6 to 12,000 live births, occurring more frequently on the right side and slightly more frequently in men.[3]

Half of microtia cases are isolated, and half are associated with other findings, most often other craniofacial anomalies. Ninety percent of microtia cases are unilateral, and the presence of bilateral microtia indicates a higher risk of other associated anomalies or an underlying syndrome.

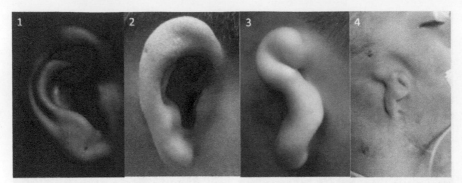

Fig. 2. Grade 1: mild malformation of the ear, with largely normal appearance. Grade 2: obvious malformation of the ear, with roughly normal size. Grade 3: complete lack of differentiation of the cartilaginous ear with developed lobe. Grade 4: lack of development of any normal external ear structure (anotia).

In most cases, microtia is a sporadic mutation with no identifiable cause. However, microtia is known to have both teratogenic and genetic triggers. The most commonly associated teratogen is isotretinoin, which has also been associated with a wide array of other congenital defects. More recent data have also suggested an increase in microtia in children born to mothers with perinatal alcohol or methamphetamine use.[4,5]

The genetic basis for microtia continues to be poorly understood, and it has been reported that only small minority of microtia cases have a hereditary basis.[3] The most common hereditary cause is Treacher Collins syndrome (TCS), which is also

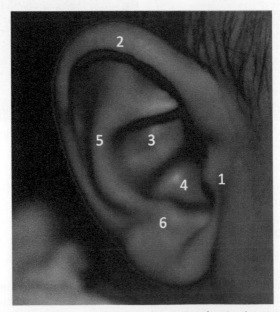

Fig. 3. Normal ear landmarks. 1: Tragus; 2: Helix; 3: Concha Cymba; 4: Concha Cavum; 5: Antihelix; 6: Antihelix.

notable for its autosomal dominant inheritance pattern. Severity and laterality of microtia in subsequent children is not predictable at this time.

SURGICAL INDICATIONS/CONTRAINDICATIONS IN MICROTIA

The indication for surgical correction of microtia includes both cosmetic and functional rehabilitation and the attendant psychosocial concerns associated with a significant facial difference. Functional aspects of the outer ear include the ability to support eyeglasses and hearing aids for the small number who are candidates for conventional hearing aids.

SURGICAL TECHNIQUE/PROCEDURE: MICROTIA REPAIR

Auricular reconstruction is a topic that continues to challenge reconstructive surgeons. Although observation (nonintervention) and prosthetics are acceptable forms of management, there are 2 broadly practiced paradigms of microtia reconstruction: (1) autologous rib cartilage–based reconstruction and (2) alloplastic reconstruction with high-density porous polyethylene. Autologous cartilage–based reconstruction continues to be the most widely practiced surgical method. In a survey of the American Society of Plastic Surgeons, cartilage microtia reconstruction was practiced by 91% of respondents and used exclusively by 70% of respondents.[6]

AUTOLOGOUS MICROTIA RECONSTRUCTION

Rib cartilage–based auricular reconstruction has been practiced in its modern form since the late 1950s.[7]

Burt Brent and Satoru Nagata popularized the 2 major techniques that have dominated microtia reconstruction for decades. Although both techniques continue to be widely practiced, multiple evolutions of the techniques have occurred.[8–12] The key features and steps of each technique are shown in **Table 1**).[13]

BRENT TECHNIQUE

The principle advantage of the Brent technique is that a smaller volume of cartilage is required and, as such, reconstruction can be started at a younger age. Most frequently reconstruction starts at age 6 or 7 years. The main disadvantage is that multiple stages are required.

The Nagata technique involves a larger volume of cartilage and is, therefore, deferred until age 10 years. Further, projection away from the skull using the Nagata method relies on placement of a projection block behind the cartilage frame, which is lined with temporoparietal fascia, harvested simultaneously with the second stage.

Table 1	
Brent and Nagata microtia reconstruction techniques	
Brent Technique	**Nagata Technique**
Creation and implantation of the rib framework (**Fig. 4**)	Creation of the entire auricular framework (**Fig. 6**)
Transposition of the lobule (**Fig. 5**)	Elevation and creation of a postauricular sulcus
Elevation and creation of postauricular sulcus	
Creation of a tragus and ensuring frontal symmetry	

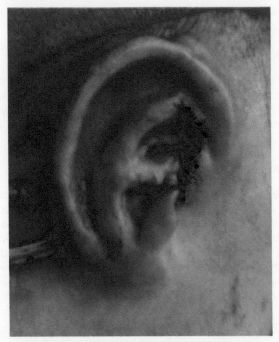

Fig. 4. Brent technique stage 1: cartilage framework creation and implantation.

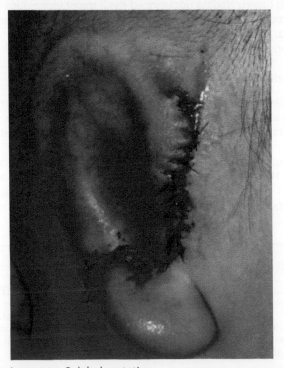

Fig. 5. Brent technique stage 2: lobule rotation.

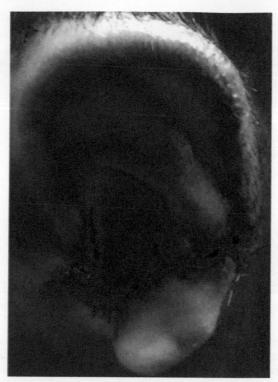

Fig. 6. Nagata technique stage 1: cartilage framework creation including tragus and implantation, lobule rotation.

Although the advantage of the Nagata technique is that it is performed in fewer stages, each of the 2 stages is more extensive. The other disadvantage is that the repair needs to be deferred until a later age.

Typical Brent and Nagata style frameworks can be seen in **Fig. 7.**

Results from reconstruction of Grade 2 (**Fig. 8**) and Grade 3 (**Fig. 9**) microtia are shown.

ALLOPLASTIC RECONSTRUCTION

The use of a synthetic, preformed auricular implant covered with autologous soft tissue was first pursued in the early 1980s. Since that time, multiple evolutions of this technique have occurred. The distinct advantages of this approach are that it can generally be accomplished in 1 or 2 stages and the donor site morbidity associated with rib cartilage harvest can be avoided. Reconstruction can also be performed as young as 3 years.[14–17] The primary disadvantages are the long-term use of a foreign implant with a higher rate of implant exposure rate, scalp alopecia, and an unnatural feel of the ear compared with rib graft.[18]

FACIAL ANOMALIES ASSOCIATED WITH MICROTIA

Microtia can be found in isolation but is commonly associated with other facial anomalies as well as multiple syndromes. Hemifacial microsomia is one of the major diagnoses affiliated with microtia with an incidence of 1:5600 live births.[19] An

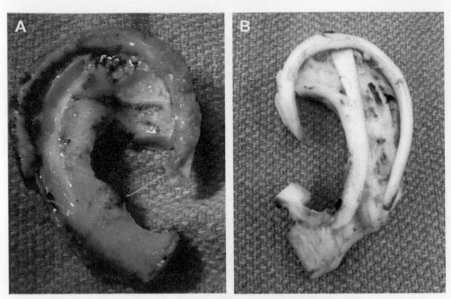

Fig. 7. (A) Brent style cartilage framework; (B) Nagata style cartilage framework.

underdevelopment of one side of the face including both the bony structures as well as the soft tissues is the definition of hemifacial microsomia. Mandibular deformity and deficiency is present and temporomandibular joint (TMJ) abnormalities may be found. Middle and inner ear structures may also be absent or malformed.

Goldenhar syndrome (GS), which is better described as oculo-auriculo-vertebral syndrome, has hemifacial microsomia and microtia as 2 of the cardinal features (**Figs. 10** and **11**). GS is a spectrum of anomalies involving the first and second branchial arches. Cardinal features are listed in **Table 2**. Although autosomal dominance can be found in these cases, many are sporadic or autosomal recessive. There is a 3:2 male and right-sided predilection. The incidence is variable with a range of 1:3500 to 25,000 births. Microtia is found in 65% of cases of GS and findings may be bilateral in as many as one-third of cases.[1,20]

TCS, also known as mandibulofacial dysostosis, can have autosomal dominant inheritance although most cases are sporadic (60%). The incidence is 1:50,000 births and is frequently associated with the TCOF1 gene although other genes have been implicated.[21,22] The primary clinical features of TCS are listed in **Table 3**. TCS is also related to anomalies of the first and second branchial arches and shares many of the features of hemifacial microsomia but presents with bilateral and frequently symmetric deformity. Microtia is a very common finding in TCS (60% of cases) and 30% also have aural atresia. Ocular deformities are often present (ie, down-sloping palpebral fissures and lower eyelid colobomas) and may require surgical intervention. Maxillary and mandibular hypoplasias are also common findings and some patients will have cleft lip and/or palate, short palate, and choanal atresia (**Fig. 12**).[1]

Nager syndrome (NS), acrofacial dysostosis, is very similar in presentation to TCS. See **Fig. 13**. However, additional preaxial limb anomalies (ie, hypoplastic thumb, radius, and humerus) are also present. Up to 80% of patients with NS have microtia.[23] Facial anomalies are similar to that found in TCS. As NS is rare, most cases of NS occur due to a spontaneous mutation without Mendelian inheritance. However, in

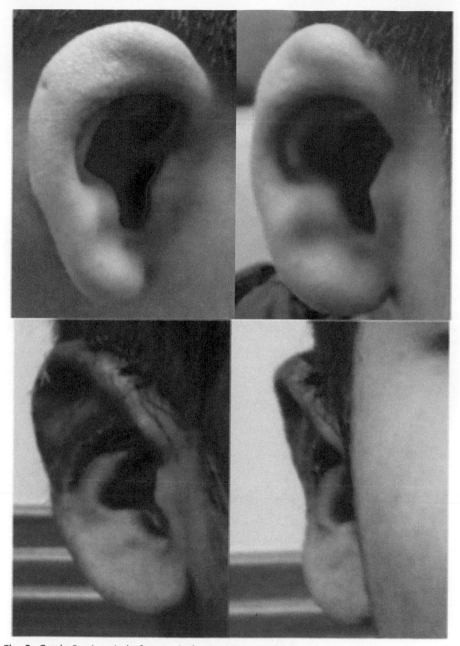

Fig. 8. Grade 2 microtia before and after reconstruction.

more recent studies, an associated gene, SF3B4, has been identified in patients pre-senting with an autosomal dominant inheritance pattern.[24,25] Some patients with NS have cardiac anomalies in addition to the craniofacial and limb anomalies. These car-diac findings are more often found with the SF3B4 mutation, which is also involved in heart development.[26]

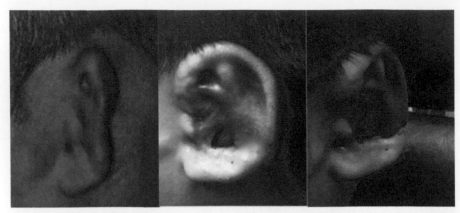

Fig. 9. Grade 3 microtia before and after reconstruction.

Macrostomia is a type of facial cleft (Tessier type 7) that is commonly associated with microtia and preauricular skin appendages (**Fig. 14**). The incidence is 1:80,000 live births.[27] In addition, 2.5% of patients with microtia also have macrostomia. Many patients with macrostomia will require treatment for oral incompetence and facial deformity. However, mild forms may not require surgical intervention.

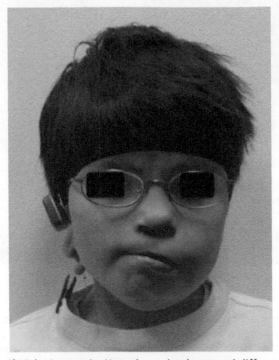

Fig. 10. Right hemifacial microsomia. Note the occlusal cant and difference of orbital position with right microtia.

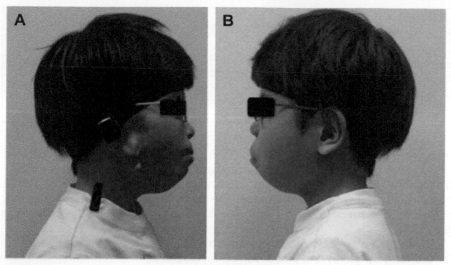

Fig. 11. Hemifacial microsomia. (*A*) Affected side with microtia; (*B*) unaffected side.

SURGICAL INDICATIONS/CONTRAINDICATIONS IN FACIAL ANOMALIES: MANDIBULAR RECONSTRUCTION

The mandible may grow insufficiently due to intrinsic causes (such as what is found in TCS, NS, and hemifacial microsomia). However, growth deficiency may also occur due to extrinsic causes. This is most notable in Pierre Robin sequence where "catch up growth" may occur and surgical intervention may not be required.[28]

The spectrum of mandibular deformities is described by the Pruzansky-Kaban classification system in **Box 1**. When mandibular asymmetry is noted to be persistent and significant based on clinical and radiographic findings, surgical intervention is indicated.

The timing of intervention will depend on the severity of symptoms. These may include obstructive sleep apnea (OSA), severe facial deformity, and malocclusion. However, indications for surgical intervention in the milder deformities (such as Pruzansky-Kaban types I and IIa) can be harder to define and delaying intervention into adolescence should be considered. According to the meta-analysis by Plomp and colleagues[22] in 2016, there is no evidence that OSA symptoms will naturally improve with time in TCS, which may be applied to other similar syndromes and congenital deformities. Therefore, when symptoms and objective evidence support OSA, an intervention of some type is indicated.

Mandibular deficiency often affects the airway by causing tongue base prolapse, which results in oropharyngeal obstruction. As a result, special consideration must be taken for airway management in the perioperative period for these patients. Intubation may require advanced techniques and in some cases tracheostomy will be

Table 2	
Clinical features of Goldenhar/oculo-auriculo-vertebral syndrome	
Hemifacial microsomia	Both autosomal recessive and autosomal dominant
Epibulbar (eye) dermoid	Microtia
Macrostomia	Vertebral malformations

Table 3 Clinical features of Treacher Collins syndrome	
Midface hypoplasia	Normal to above normal intelligence
Downward-sloping palpebral fissures	*Autosomal dominant (40% of cases)*
Micrognathia/Retrognathia	Conductive hearing loss
Lower eyelid abnormalities	Cleft palate
Microtia	Choanal atresia

required.[29] Up to 37% of patients with NS will require tracheostomy as an infant, and mortality has been reported at 12% due to respiratory issues.[23] Mandibular distraction osteogenesis (MDO) in patients with TCS and NS for airway improvement should, however, be considered with caution as some reports have shown limited growth after completion of distraction and in some cases a return to the preoperative position was the result.[30,31]

Mandibular distraction for unilateral deformity has been shown to be very effective for providing symmetry and proper occlusion specifically in patients with hemifacial microsomia. A study by Weichmann published in 2017 looked at their results over a 21-year period and found the best, most reliable and consistent results in those patients with mild to moderate deformity (Pruzansky-Kaban I–IIa).[32] The average age for intervention in their study was 5½ years.

A meta-analysis by Pluijmers and colleagues[33] in 2014 also looked at unilateral MDO and concurred that reliable, long-standing results can be achieved in mild deformity as a single-stage technique; however, surgical correction of more severe mandibular deformities should be considered as a multi-stage treatment protocol. Whichever technique is pursued, both functional as well as psychological benefits have been consistently encountered.

As with any surgery, complications occasionally happen with mandibular surgery. In addition to airway concerns, injury to neurologic and dental structures can occur. Most injuries are transient although permanent injury may occur.

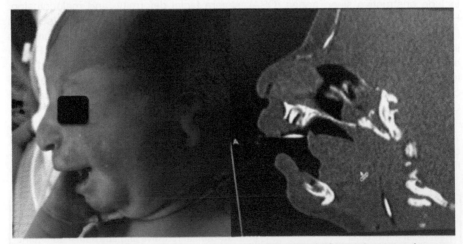

Fig. 12. Patient with Treacher Collins syndrome. Note retrognathia with tongue base prolapse and choanal atresia noted on computed tomographic (CT) scan. Patient also has microtia but no cleft palate.

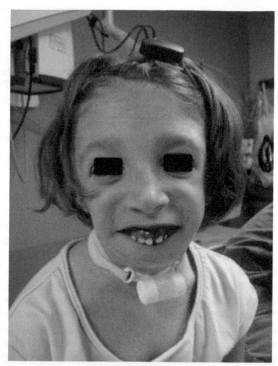

Fig. 13. Patient with Nager syndrome. Note tracheostomy related to OSA from retrognathia. Other findings are deficient soft palate without cleft palate and overdeveloped maxilla.

SURGICAL TECHNIQUE/PROCEDURE AND OUTCOMES: MANDIBULAR SURGERY

Depending on the deformity, different surgical techniques can be used for mandibular reconstruction, which can involve a more standard advancement (with or without

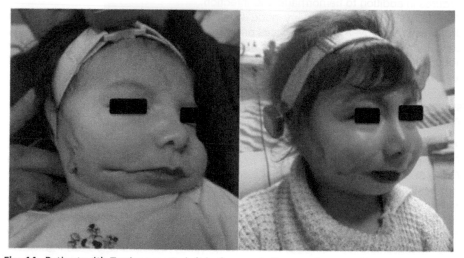

Fig. 14. Patient with Tessier type 7 cleft before and after repair.

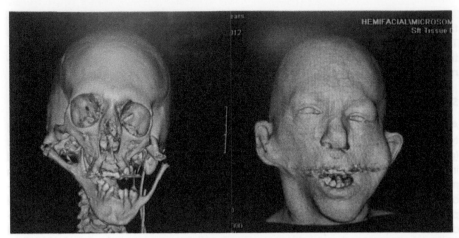

Fig. 16. CT scan 3D reconstruction of adult patient with GS including epibulbar dermoid, bilateral hemifacial microsomia. Note progressive distortion with asymmetry.

computed tomographic (CT) scan and physical examination confirm obstruction at the oropharynx and nasopharyngeal level and external deformity is significant.

Distraction osteogenesis is usually used for severe discrepancy and multivector movement, whereas less severe issues can be treated with maxillary advancement with rigid fixation.

Most cases of microtia do not include periorbital deformity or at least do not require surgical intervention for the mild deformities. However, in cases of severe deformity, where the bony orbital rim is incomplete, such as is commonly found in TCS and NS, surgery may be elected to provide support to the globe and the periorbital tissues. The age at intervention is important to consider because bony resorption has been found to be very high in patients undergoing surgery before age 5 years (up to 99%) and least (14%) in those who are 13 years or older at the time of intervention.[34] Many choose to intervene at approximately age 7 years expecting an acceptable 25% resorption rate for the grafts.

If inorganic materials are selected for malar and orbital reconstruction, there is a greater chance of infection and dislocation compared with autologous graft materials.[35,36]

Eyelid deformities (ie, malposition of the canthi and coloboma) can also be performed when necessary. Indications for intervention include xerophthalmia (dry eyes) and exposure keratopathy in addition to morphologic deformity. Patients with TCS often have coloboma of the eyelid and when it involves greater than one-third of the eyelid, the likelihood of needing surgery in infancy is much greater.[22] When the visual axis is at risk, excision of the epibulbar limbal dermoid (commonly found in GS) is recommended as early as 3 months of age.[37]

SURGICAL TECHNIQUE/PROCEDURE AND OUTCOMES: MAXILLARY AND ORBITAL RECONSTRUCTION

Periorbital skeletal surgery may be approached as an isolated procedure or in coordination with maxillary surgery. A transconjunctival or a subciliary incision (both being around the eye) can be used for the approach although a bicoronal incision (which is up on the scalp) may allow for bilateral intervention without periorbital incisions.[25]

Split calvarial bone or rib can be selected for autologous grafting although prosthetics can be generated using preoperative CT guidance and used successfully. This surgery is ideally performed at or after age 7 years when bony maturation is close to complete.[38]

The soft tissue work on the eyelid and periorbita may use z-plasty techniques or wedge excisions. When there is tissue deficiency causing exposure problems, full-thickness skin grafts can be added from areas such as the postauricular skin or from the lower neck.

SURGICAL INDICATIONS/CONTRAINDICATIONS IN FACIAL ANOMALIES: MACROSTOMIA REPAIR

The Tessier type 7 cleft lip, macrostomia, frequently occurs ipsilateral to the patient's side with microtia. Macrostomia is most commonly unilateral, but it can occur bilaterally with varying degrees of severity. Skin tags are often present as well. In mild cases, surgery may not be pursued. However, when obvious deformity is apparent and/or oral incompetence is present, surgical repair is indicated. Risks associated with this surgery are similar to any surgical repair of facial soft tissues and should be done after 3 months of age.

SURGICAL TECHNIQUE/PROCEDURE AND OUTCOMES: MACROSTOMIA REPAIR

Similar to more typical cleft lips, the Tessier type 7 cleft presents as a partial or complete discontinuity of the orbicularis oris muscle and lateralization of the oral commissure (see **Fig. 14**). The other muscles of facial expression are often hypoplastic with inappropriate attachments. The surgical plan should include correction of the location and attachments of the facial muscles affected in addition to the reconstruction of the orbicularis oris muscle and reconstitution of the oral commissure. When used correctly, a symmetric and competent mouth opening can be achieved (see **Fig. 14**).

The principles of reconstruction involve repair of all 3 soft tissue layers, including mucosa, muscle, and skin. Multiple surgical techniques have been described with each one aiming at achieving the ideal muscle position. Thus, a natural position to the commissure can be created both in repose as well as in active position. A Z-plasty or W-plasty at the melolabial fold is commonly performed to reduce scar contracture and allow for better positioning of the commissure although some studies have refuted the necessity of anything besides a straight-line closure.[27,39]

SUMMARY

Microtia is an easily identifiable malformation of the external ear caused by a malformation of the first and second branchial arches. Although microtia occurs in isolation 50% of the time, there can be many associated craniofacial or systemic anomalies. The identification of microtia and associated facial anomalies can help guide perinatal care providers toward a unifying diagnosis. This can result in earlier diagnosis of disease and allow for a more streamlined approach to diagnosis, consultation, and management of affected patients.

With advances in microtia and craniofacial reconstruction, the outlook for these patients is positive and outcomes continue to improve. However, the surgical correction of these anomalies is complex and must be thoughtfully integrated into the overall care plan, which can also be complex in these patients.

REFERENCES

1. Wetmore R, Muntz H, McGill T. Pediatric otolaryngology: principles and practice pathways. 2nd edition. New York: Thieme; 2012.
2. Vincent C, Kalatzis V, Abdelhak S, et al. BOR and BO syndromes are allelic defects of EYA1. Eur J Hum Genet 1997;5(4):242–6.
3. Klockars T, Rautio J. Embryology and epidemiology of microtia. Facial Plast Surg 2009;25(3):145–8.
4. Forrester MB, Merz RD. Risk of selected birth defects with prenatal illicit drug use, Hawaii, 1986-2002. J Toxicol Environ Health A 2007;70(1):7–18.
5. Jahn AF, Ganti K. Major auricular malformations due to Accutane (isotretinoin). Laryngoscope 1987;97(7 Pt 1):832–5.
6. Im DD, Paskhover B, Staffenberg DA, et al. Current management of microtia: a national survey. Aesthetic Plast Surg 2013;37(2):402–8.
7. TANZER RC. Total reconstruction of the external ear. Plast Reconstr Surg Transplant Bull 1959;23(1):1–15.
8. Firmin F. Ear reconstruction in cases of typical microtia. Personal experience based on 352 microtic ear corrections. Scand J Plast Reconstr Surg Hand Surg 1998;32(1):35–47.
9. Firmin F. State-of-the-art autogenous ear reconstruction in cases of microtia. Adv Otorhinolaryngol 2010;68:25–52.
10. Firmin F, Marchac A. A novel algorithm for autologous ear reconstruction. Semin Plast Surg 2011;25(4):257–64.
11. Kasrai L, Snyder-Warwick AK, Fisher DM. Single-stage autologous ear reconstruction for microtia. Plast Reconstr Surg 2014;133(3):652–62.
12. Park C. Discussion: single-stage autologous ear reconstruction for microtia. Plast Reconstr Surg 2014;133(3):663–5.
13. Yotsuyanagi T, Yamashita K, Yamauchi M, et al. Correction of lobule-type microtia: I. The first stage of costal cartilage grafting. Plast Reconstr Surg 2014;133(1):111–20.
14. Berghaus A. Porecon implant and fan flap: a concept for reconstruction of the auricle. Facial Plast Surg 1988;5(5):451–7.
15. Wellisz T. Clinical experience with the Medpor porous polyethylene implant. Aesthetic Plast Surg 1993;17(4):339–44.
16. Reinisch JF, Lewin S. Ear reconstruction using a porous polyethylene framework and temporoparietal fascia flap. Facial Plast Surg 2009;25(3):181–9.
17. Yang SL, Zheng JH, Ding Z, et al. Combined fascial flap and expanded skin flap for enveloping Medpor framework in microtia reconstruction. Aesthetic Plast Surg 2009;33(4):518–22.
18. Romo T, Morris LG, Reitzen SD, et al. Reconstruction of congenital microtia-atresia: outcomes with the Medpor/bone-anchored hearing aid-approach. Ann Plast Surg 2009;62(4):384–9.
19. Wolford LM, Perez DE. Surgical management of congenital deformities with temporomandibular joint malformation. Oral Maxillofac Surg Clin North Am 2015;27(1):137–54.
20. Gorlin R, Cohen M, Levin L. Branchial arch and oro-acral disorders. New York: Oxford; 1990.
21. Tse WK. Treacher Collins syndrome: new insights from animal models. Int J Biochem Cell Biol 2016;81(Pt A):44–7.
22. Plomp RG, van Lieshout MJ, Joosten KF, et al. Treacher Collins syndrome: a systematic review of evidence-based treatment and recommendations. Plast Reconstr Surg 2016;137(1):191–204.

23. Herrmann BW, Karzon R, Molter DW. Otologic and audiologic features of Nager acrofacial dysostosis. Int J Pediatr Otorhinolaryngol 2005;69(8):1053–9.
24. Bernier FP, Caluseriu O, Ng S, et al. Haploinsufficiency of SF3B4, a component of the pre-mRNA spliceosomal complex, causes Nager syndrome. Am J Hum Genet 2012;90(5):925–33.
25. Chummun S, McLean NR, Anderson PJ, et al. The craniofacial and upper limb management of Nager syndrome. J Craniofac Surg 2016;27(4):932–7.
26. Ruiz-Lozano P, Doevendans P, Brown A, et al. Developmental expression of the murine spliceosome-associated protein mSAP49. Dev Dyn 1997;208(4):482–90.
27. Rogers GF, Mulliken JB. Repair of transverse facial cleft in hemifacial microsomia: long-term anthropometric evaluation of commissural symmetry. Plast Reconstr Surg 2007;120(3):728–37.
28. Daskalogiannakis J, Ross RB, Tompson BD. The mandibular catch-up growth controversy in Pierre Robin sequence. Am J Orthod Dentofacial Orthop 2001; 120(3):280–5.
29. Perkins JA, Sie KC, Milczuk H, et al. Airway management in children with craniofacial anomalies. Cleft Palate Craniofac J 1997;34(2):135–40.
30. Anderson PJ, Netherway DJ, Abbott A, et al. Mandibular lengthening by distraction for airway obstruction in treacher-collins syndrome: the long-term results. J Craniofac Surg 2004;15(1):47–50.
31. Stelnicki EJ, Lin WY, Lee C, et al. Long-term outcome study of bilateral mandibular distraction: a comparison of Treacher Collins and Nager syndromes to other types of micrognathia. Plast Reconstr Surg 2002;109(6):1819–25 [discussion: 1826–7].
32. Weichman KE, Jacobs J, Patel P, et al. Early distraction for mild to moderate unilateral craniofacial microsomia: long-term follow-up, outcomes, and recommendations. Plast Reconstr Surg 2017;139(4):941e–53e.
33. Pluijmers BI, Caron CJ, Dunaway DJ, et al. Mandibular reconstruction in the growing patient with unilateral craniofacial microsomia: a systematic review. Int J Oral Maxillofac Surg 2014;43(3):286–95.
34. Fan KL, Federico C, Kawamoto HK, et al. Optimizing the timing and technique of Treacher Collins orbital malar reconstruction. J Craniofac Surg 2012;23(7 Suppl 1):2033–7.
35. Chrcanovic BR, Abreu MH. Survival and complications of zygomatic implants: a systematic review. Oral Maxillofac Surg 2013;17(2):81–93.
36. Chrcanovic BR, Albrektsson T, Wennerberg A. Survival and complications of zygomatic implants: an updated systematic review. J Oral Maxillofac Surg 2016;74(10): 1949–64.
37. Panda A, Ghose S, Khokhar S, et al. Surgical outcomes of Epibulbar dermoids. J Pediatr Ophthalmol Strabismus 2002;39(1):20–5.
38. Galea CJ, Dashow JE, Woerner JE. Congenital abnormalities of the temporomandibular joint. Oral Maxillofac Surg Clin North Am 2018;30(1):71–82.
39. Kajikawa A, Ueda K, Katsuragi Y, et al. Surgical repair of transverse facial cleft: oblique vermilion-mucosa incision. J Plast Reconstr Aesthet Surg 2010;63(8): 1269–74.

Identification and Management of Cranial Anomalies in Perinatology

James D. Vargo, MD[a], Ayesha Hasan, MD[b],
Brian T. Andrews, MD[a,c],*

KEYWORDS

- Cranial anomaly • Prenatal diagnosis • Cranial malformation • Head shape deformity
- Craniosynostosis • Deformational plagiocephaly

KEY POINTS

- Craniosynostosis and deformational plagiocephaly are the most commonly encountered cranial anomalies. Cutis aplasia and encephalocele are seen less frequently.
- Improvements in prenatal imaging have allowed improved and earlier detection of rare cranial anomalies.
- Abnormal cranial morphology can be visualized on prenatal ultrasonography as early as the second trimester, although cranial sutures cannot be readily seen. Imaging should also assess for limb, skeletal, and cerebral anomalies.
- Suspicion for a craniosynostosis syndrome based on family history and/or findings on imaging may indicate further investigation with amniocentesis for common genetic mutations.
- Management of cranial anomalies requires a multidisciplinary approach, starting with the perinatologist.

INTRODUCTION

Cranial malformations and congenital head shape anomalies are common, with one study showing an incidence as high as 24.6%.[1] Cranial malformations present with a broad spectrum of phenotypes as well as great variation in severity, making

Disclosures: None of the authors of this article have any commercial or financial conflicts of interest or sources of funding to disclose.
[a] Department of Plastic Surgery, University of Kansas Medical Center, 3901 Rainbow Boulevard, Kansas City, KS 66160, USA; [b] Department of Obstetrics and Gynecology, University of Kansas Medical Center, 3901 Rainbow Boulevard, Kansas City, KS 66160, USA; [c] Department of Otolaryngology–Head and Neck Surgery, University of Kansas Medical Center, 3901 Rainbow Boulevard, Kansas City, KS 66160, USA
* Corresponding author. Department of Plastic Surgery, University of Kansas Medical Center, 3901 Rainbow Boulevard, Kansas City, KS 66160.
E-mail address: bandrews@kumc.edu

Clin Perinatol 45 (2018) 699–715
https://doi.org/10.1016/j.clp.2018.07.008
0095-5108/18/© 2018 Elsevier Inc. All rights reserved.

epidemiologic studies difficult to conduct and interpret. Recent advances in prenatal imaging, including three-dimensional (3D) ultrasonography, computed tomography (CT), and fetal MRI (fMRI), have provided better means of early detection of head shape anomalies in utero.[2] As such, perinatologists have become increasingly involved in the diagnosis and management of neonates with cranial anomalies and, as such, should be considered the gatekeepers for prenatal care and parental counseling.

There are several conditions that most frequently affect the neonatal skull. Most cases fit within the spectrum of 2 conditions: craniosynostosis (CS) and deformational plagiocephaly (DP). Other less common cranial anomalies include cutis aplasia and encephalocele. An understanding of the pathophysiology involved in each condition is important because phenotypes can be similar, causing confusion and misdiagnosis. Accurate early diagnosis is essential because treatments vary greatly depending on the diagnosis, ranging from nonoperative interventions to intracranial surgery. Delays in accurate diagnosis can affect both aesthetic and developmental outcomes for newborns with cranial anomalies.

Cranial Development

Neonatal cranial development begins during the third or fourth week of gestation via formation of 7 bones that become the cranial vault (paired frontal, parietal, and temporal bones, and a single occipital bone). Between each bone is a cranial suture that is a synarthrosis, or fibrous joint. Cranial sutures are the location of most new bone deposition and cranial growth during early skull development. Cranial bone growth occurs primarily in response to increasing brain size and cerebrospinal fluid volume, which initiates a complex signaling pathway between the dura and suture mesenchymal cells.[3] because sutures are linear structures, cranial bones grow primarily perpendicular to these sites of ossification (Virchow's law).[4] This process occurs rapidly in infants, with the brain and skull tripling in size by 1 year and reaching 85% of adult volume at 3 years. By age 6 to 10 years, the skull is near adult size.[5] In addition, cranial sutures also function to permit some degree of deformation during delivery, allowing the fetal skull to pass through the birth canal without trauma.[6] Sutures close at predictable times during development, occurring from anterior to posterior. The metopic suture typically closes first early within the first year of life, followed by sagittal at ~22 years, coronal at ~24 years, and lambdoid sutures at ~26 years of age. In addition, neonates have 2 fontanelles, or cranial soft spots," which close at 3 to 6 months anteriorly and posteriorly between 9 and 12 months.

CRANIOSYNOSTOSIS

CS refers to premature fusion of 1 or more of the cranial sutures. CS commences early in development with cranial suture closure beginning before birth. As a result, inappropriately fused cranial sutures restrict normal skull growth. As the brain continues to grow irrespective of the skull disorder, it becomes mechanically constrained by a noncompliant skull. This constraint forces the remaining patent sutures and areas of compliant skull to expand, creating abnormal head shapes that can be appreciated even in utero. In rare cases, the skull cannot sufficiently accommodate the rapidly growing brain, causing increase of intracranial pressure (ICP), especially when more than 1 suture is fused.[7] Persistently increased ICPs can result in neurologic dysfunction and developmental delay if not addressed surgically.

CS most commonly exists in isolation (nonsyndromic) but it can be part of a genetic syndrome such as Apert syndrome, Crouzon syndrome, Pfeiffer syndrome, Saethre-Chotzen syndrome, or Muenke syndrome.[8] The incidence of nonsyndromic CS ranges from 1:1800 to 1:2500 births,[9,10] and typically is isolated to a single cranial suture (simple CS), although multiple sutures can be involved (complex CS). The sagittal suture is most commonly involved (55% of cases), followed by metopic (24%), unilateral coronal (15%), and lambdoid sutures (4%).[11] However, the epidemiology of specific suture involvement seems to be changing, because recent studies have identified an increasing incidence of metopic CS for unknown reasons.[12] Syndromic cases of CS are much less common, are more likely to involve multiple sutures (bicoronal most frequently), and commonly have associated facial and limb anomalies.

Causes

Multiple theories exist regarding the causes of CS, and likely multiple factors are involved concurrently. The intrinsic theory cites abnormalities of the osteoinductive properties of the dura, causing cessation of cranial bone deposition.[13,14] Without new bone being formed, the cranial sutures prematurely fuse. However, the extrinsic theory proposes that factors outside the dura/suture complex induce closure via in utero compression, hydrocephalus, abnormal brain growth, or systemic diseases (rickets, hypothyroidism). Syndromic CS results from mutation of genes involved in the signaling pathway between the dura and suture mesenchyme, resulting in failure of bone production and premature closure of sutures.[15]

Pathogenesis

Premature fusion of 1 or more cranial sutures has several downstream consequences as bone growth is arrested at this portion of the calvarium. CS causes the skull to develop compensatory growth patterns typically in the direction perpendicular to any fused suture. This process creates predictable patterns of abnormal head shape based on the specific sutures involved. Abnormal cranial head shape can lead to other facial abnormalities, such as malposition of the ears, orbits, nose, and mandible. Malposition typically results from an abnormal skull base that corresponds with concomitant cranial vault anomalies.

Single-suture CS involvement rarely causes increases in ICP (17%) and therefore concerns for this condition are only warranted if other overt concomitant signs/symptoms exist.[16] However, when multiple sutures are affected, the skull volume is more likely to become restricted and the incidence of increased cranial pressure increases to nearly half of affected neonates (47%).[17] The brain grows intrinsically during infancy and continues to expand even in the setting of unequal skull growth. This craniocerebral disproportion can lead to increased ICPs, defined as borderline when greater than 15 mm Hg and pathologic when greater than 20 mm Hg. This condition can be compensated for to a degree by bulging fontanelles at the cranial vertex and bossing of nonaffected cranial bones.[18] When this mechanism fails and ICPs are persistently increased, neurologic dysfunction and developmental delays can occur.

Neurologic Development

Developmental delay and lower intelligence quotient scores occur in individuals with CS at a higher frequency than in the general population.[19] This delay is more significant when multiple sutures are affected.[20] The cause of the delay is unclear and may be related to early brain growth restriction. It is possible that the cellular and molecular process causing early cranial suture fusion also negatively affects central nervous system development. Evidence suggests that surgical repair of CS results in overall improved intelligence and those infants more than 12 months of age with delay can have improved developmental outcomes following surgery.[21] Prolonged increase of ICP can also cause papilledema and ultimately optic nerve atrophy, leading to irreversible visual impairment.[18]

DEFORMATIONAL PLAGIOCEPHALY

DP is another common neonatal cranial anomaly. Its incidence has increased over the past decade and it is seen in 1 in 300 births.[22] DP is also termed positional plagiocephaly because it results from prolonged, abnormal head positioning and compensatory external pressures, which affects cranial bone growth and head shape. These abnormal head shapes arise as the developing brain is impinged by external forces, such as the pelvis preventing growth in certain directions. More commonly, DP results after birth as a result of prolonged supine positioning during early infancy. Its incidence has greatly increased since the 1992 Back to Sleep campaign from the American Academy of Pediatrics to decrease the risk of sudden infant death syndrome (SIDS).[22–26] Although this has drastically decreased the risk of SIDS, DP has increased by 600%.[22]

In rare circumstances, DP begins in utero when the developing fetal head and cranium are compressed secondary to abnormal uterine positioning.[27] It is common for 1 or more of neonates born to mothers carrying multiples to be affected by this condition to varying degrees.[28] DP can be mistaken for CS, most frequently lambdoid synostosis, because both present with occipital flattening. The two conditions can be differentiated because lambdoid CS causes the ipsilateral ear to be positioned posteriorly, and seldom affects the forehead initially, whereas DP causes a parallelogram-shaped head with anterior positioning of the ear and ipsilateral forehead bossing.[29]

OTHER CRANIAL ANOMALIES

Cutis aplasia and encephalocele are two other rare cranial malformations that might be detected in utero. Cutis aplasia is a condition that results in the absence of the vertex scalp skin (mild cases); scalp skin and cranial bone (moderate cases); or scalp skin, bone, and dura (severe cases). Encephaloceles are congenital defects in the developing skull that allow the brain to herniate outside the cranial vault in what is often a stalklike appearance. They most commonly occur posteriorly (75%); however, anterior (sincipital) encephaloceles are considerably more deforming.[30] Anteriorly, this condition is often referred to as midline nasal masses, which results from anterior skull base defects at the foramen cecum (**Fig. 1**). In most cases, the midline nasal mass is simply trapped skin material, termed a dermoid, which forms between a closed foramen cecum and the glabellar skin. When the foramen cecum remains patent, herniating neural tissue through the anterior skull base may contain the meninges alone in mild cases, meninges and brain in moderate cases, and the meninges, brain, and part of the ventricular system in severe cases. The herniated neural tissue is commonly nonfunctional and, as such, its removal at the time of surgical correction is inconsequential to future neurodevelopment.

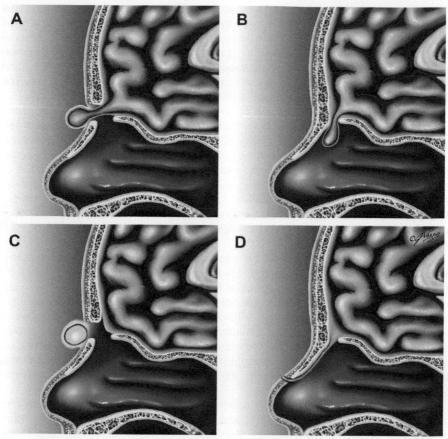

Fig. 1. (*A*) Frontal (sincipital) encephalocele including herniation through a patent fonticulus frontalis at the junction of the developing frontal and nasal bones. (*B*) Frontal encephalocele through a patent foramen cecum. (*C*) Nasal dermoid cyst. (*D*) Nasal dermoid tract with intracranial extension. (*Courtesy of* James D. Vargo, MD, Kansas City, KS.)

PRENATAL EVALUATION OF CRANIAL ANOMALIES
Risk Factors

Multiple risk factors have been implicated in causing cranial anomalies and should be considered during normal pregnancy screenings. These risk factors include multiple gestations, abnormal uterine lie, family history of CS or associated syndromes, advanced maternal age, white maternal race, gestation at high altitude, nitrosatable drug exposure, paternal occupation, and many others.[31] No single risk factor has a high correlation with development of any particular cranial anomaly. Risk factors for in utero DP include abnormal uterine position and multiple gestations. Presence of 1 or more risk factors for CS and/or DP should increase suspicion during routine prenatal evaluation.

Radiographic Imaging

Measurement of cranial growth via ultrasonography is part of routine prenatal care and provides an opportunity to evaluate head shape without additional testing or office visits. Although cranial sutures are difficult to visualize with standard prenatal ultrasonography, restricted cranial growth and abnormal morphology of the skull can be detected as early as the second trimester. Axial, sagittal, and coronal cuts should all be used to evaluate the neonatal head shape. Examination from multiple views provides a more complete assessment as well as potential identification of other skeletal anomalies that may indicate CS and an associated syndrome. The skull should initially be assessed for symmetry and contour, as well as calvarial continuity to exclude encephalocele or cutis aplasia (**Fig. 2**). Measurement of the biparietal diameter (BPD) and occipitofrontal diameter (OCD) should be recorded to allows calculation of a cephalic index (CI), which provides a numeric representation of head shape by a width/length ratio. CI is calculated using the following equation: BPD/OCD × 100. A normal CI, or mesencephaly, is between 75 and 79.9. A CI less than 75 suggests dolichocephaly, or an elongated head shape. A CI greater than 79.9 suggests brachycephaly, or a shortened or rounded head shape. Although CI provides objective measurement, it does not account for specific contour abnormalities of the skull and is less reliable than visual evaluation of skull shape.

Brain parenchyma should also be evaluated to exclude intracranial masses, which may distort the head shape. Identification of ventriculomegaly must be made with caution, given this may result from distortion of the skull shape or the intracranial structures, termed a distortional ventriculomegaly. The shape and size of the orbits can be evaluated with coronal views and may be suggestive of proptosis or exorbitism. In addition, midface hypoplasia and cleft lip/palate should be examined.[32] In addition to the anatomy of the head, a thorough assessment of fetal hands, feet, and heart must be performed. Imaging of the extremities may show simple or complex syndactyly, as well as other limb anomalies that may help identify a genetic syndrome.

Ultrasonography findings typically become more pronounced as the pregnancy progresses and the head enlarges. Structures can be more easily seen on 3D or four-dimensional ultrasonography images, if available. However, abnormal head shape on ultrasonography is not sufficient for a diagnosis of CS, because positional DP in utero or misidentification of a normal head shape also frequently occur. When indicated for investigation of intracranial or other congenital anomalies, fMRI can also be used for further assessment of sutural closure; however, fMRI is rarely indicated for CS alone.

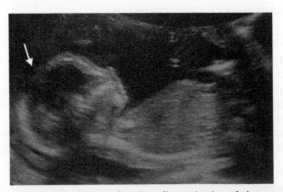

Fig. 2. Sagittal ultrasonography image showing discontinuity of the cranial vault (*arrow*), suspicious for cutis aplasia. This patient was born with cutis aplasia involving agenesis of the vertex scalp skin, subcutaneous tissue, and underlying skull.

However, the rate of detection of prenatal CS is low. A study in 2015 evaluated all cases of nonsyndromic CS between 1996 and 2012 at a high-volume tertiary medical center (n = 618 births) and found only 2 cases (0.3%) that were diagnosed prenatally.[11] Other studies have reported a rate as high as 11%.[33] Prenatal imaging is also not highly specific, as shown by a study by Fjortoft and colleagues,[34] who followed 15 patients with suspected CS based on sonographic evidence. This study reported that only 4 of the 15 (27%) neonates were diagnosed with CS postnatally. The remaining subjects were diagnosed with DP (n = 2) or were normal (n = 8). Physician skills, experience, and expertise play a major part accurate in utero identification.

Cranial Morphology

The morphology of prenatal CS mirrors the patterns seen in newborns and children with the condition and can often be identified on prenatal imaging. Sagittal CS results in scaphocephaly (boat-shaped head), with a narrowed bitemporal diameter as a result of decreased growth perpendicular to the sagittal suture (**Fig. 3**). Compensatory growth occurs in the perpendicular vector, resulting in anteroposterior elongation with frontal bossing and an occipital bulge. Metopic CS causes development of trigonocephaly (keel-shaped head), or a triangular shape to the frontal skull with bitemporal narrowing and associated orbital hypotelorism. Unilateral coronal CS commonly causes brachycephaly (short head), ipsilateral forehead flattening with contralateral frontal bossing, and ipsilateral deviation of the nasal root and chin (**Fig. 4**). Bicoronal CS also causes brachycephaly, often more severe than unilateral, along with a broad and flat forehead, wide bitemporal diameter, and elevation of skull height. In addition, lambdoid CS results in a trapezoid-shaped head with occipital flatness, ipsilateral mastoid bulge, posterior position of the ipsilateral ear, and rarely compensatory contour irregularities of the forehead.

Complex CS involving multiple sutures can present with a wide range of cranial morphologies and abnormal cranial contours. Most commonly, this presents as significant brachycephaly or turribrachycephaly when both coronal sutures are fused. When all cranial sutures are fused prematurely, the skull can take on a cloverleaf or

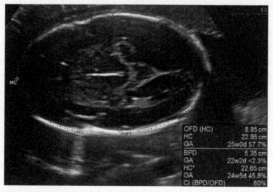

Fig. 3. Axial window on prenatal ultrasonography at 24 weeks' gestation. Although cranial sutures are not clearly defined, the scaphocephalic head shape is visible. The CI is 60, which is abnormal (normal = 75–79.9). Based on skull morphology, sagittal CS can be suspected.

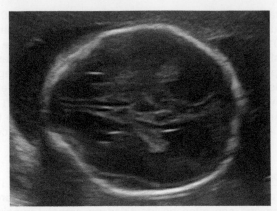

Fig. 4. Axial window on prenatal ultrasonography at 21 weeks' gestation. This neonate has a brachycephalic skull morphology and CI of 84 (normal = 75–79.9), with potential left frontal flattening and right frontal bossing, suspicious for left unicoronal or complex CS. Other findings included significant cerebral anomalies with partial Dandy-Walker malformation.

kleeblattschädel skull shape (**Fig. 5**). In this condition, the fontanelles are often significantly enlarged to relieve ICP and allow for compensatory developing brain growth.

Craniosynostosis Syndromes

An appreciation for the congenital syndromes commonly associated with CS is an important part of prenatal evaluation. This appreciation can guide both prenatal and postnatal management of these complex infants. There are more than 60 genes and 150 syndromes associated with CS. The most commonly encountered syndromes include Apert syndrome, Crouzon syndrome, Pfeiffer syndrome, Saethre-Chotzen syndrome, and Muenke syndrome[35] (**Table 1**). The constellation of presenting anomalies for each of these syndromes may be recognizable on prenatal imaging.

Apert syndrome or acrocephalosyndactyly (1:70,000) is an autosomal dominant (AD) condition associated with a mutation in the FGFR-2 receptor, which is associated with the dural-suture signaling pathway.[36] It is commonly associated with bicoronal CS, midface hypoplasia, proptosis, hypertelorism, and downslanting palpebral fissures.[37] An isolated cleft palate without cleft lip is seen in 30% of neonates. Bilateral symmetric syndactyly of the hands is characteristic for Apert syndrome. Crouzon syndrome (1:25,000) is also an AD condition associated with mutation of FGFR-2.[8] These patients commonly have brachycephaly secondary to bicoronal CS, midface hypoplasia, and proptosis.[38] Crouzon syndrome does not present with anomalies of the hands or feet, distinguishing it from some of the other CS syndromes. Pfeiffer syndrome (1:65,000–100,000) is inherited AD and can be associated with FGFR-1 or FGFR-2, which plays a role in phenotypic findings of the patient.[8] These patients typically have multisuture CS, most commonly bicoronal, and in severe cases can present with a cloverleaf or kleeblattschädel skull.[39] This finding can be seen on prenatal ultrasonography and strongly indicates Pfeiffer syndrome (see **Fig. 5**). Pfeiffer syndrome is also associated with midface hypoplasia, proptosis, and cleft palate. Broad thumbs and toes are

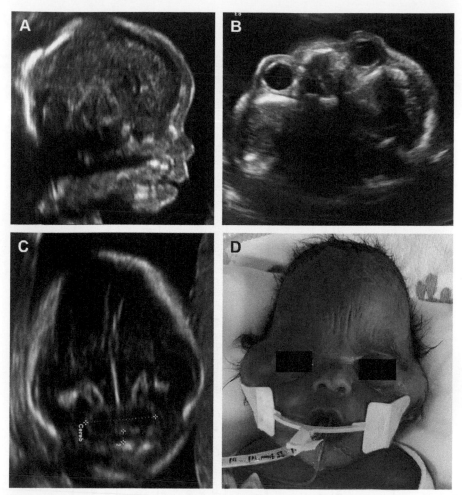

Fig. 5. Ultrasonography examination at 30 weeks' gestation and postnatal view of pansutural CS with cloverleaf or kleeblattschädel head shape. This patient was later diagnosed with Beare-Stevenson syndrome. (*A*) Sagittal cut showing abnormal midface development and cranial contour with sutural overlap. (*B*) Axial window through the orbits with significant hypertelorism and exorbitism. (*C*) Transcerebellar window showing abnormal cranial contour with bilateral temporal bulging and anterior narrowing. (*D*) Postnatal view of severe cloverleaf head shape, midface hypoplasia, hypertelorism, and exorbitism.

characteristic, and these infants can also present with simple syndactyly. Saethre-Chotzen syndrome (1:25,000–50:000) is an AD inherited mutation of the TWIST-1 gene, and can present with either unilateral or bicoronal CS, midface hypoplasia, eyelid ptosis, and prominent crura of the ear.[40] Simple syndactyly can also be seen in these infants. Muenke syndrome (1:30,000) is inherited AD and associated with a mutation of the FGFR-3 gene.[41] These patients can present with variable unilateral or bicoronal CS, midface hypoplasia, hypertelorism, downslanting palpebral fissures, and high arched palate. These patients may have brachydactyly or clinodactyly of the fingers.

Table 1
Syndromic craniosynostosis syndromes

Syndrome	Genetic Mutation	Incidence	Cranial Morphology	Midface	Hands/Feet	Neurocognitive Impairment
Apert syndrome	FGFR-2	1:70,000	Bicoronal CS	Hypertelorism, exorbitism, midface hypoplasia, downslanting palpebral fissures, isolated cleft lip/palate (30%)	Bilateral symmetric complex brachysyndactyly (thumb or small finger may be free)	Severe delay
Crouzon syndrome	FGFR-2	1:25,000	Bicoronal CS	Hypertelorism, exorbitism, midface hypoplasia, mandibular prognathism	None	Normal or mild delay
Pfeiffer syndrome	FGFR-1 (5%) FGFR-2 (95%)	1:65,000–100,000	Type 1: bicoronal CS. Type 2: moderate pansuture CS with cloverleaf skull. Type 3: severe pansuture CS with cloverleaf skull	Hypertelorism, exorbitism, midface hypoplasia, cleft palate	Broad thumbs and great toes. Simple syndactyly	Type 1: normal. Type 2/3: intellectual delay
Saethre-Chotzen syndrome	TWIST-1	1:25,000–50,000	Unilateral or bicoronal CS	Midface hypoplasia, lid ptosis, prominent ear crura, low frontal hairline	Simple syndactyly	Normal or mild delay
Muenke syndrome	FGFR-3	1:30,000	Unilateral or bicoronal CS, macrocephaly	Hypertelorism, exorbitism, midface hypoplasia, high arched palate	Brachydactyly, clinodactyly	Developmental delay

Prenatal Diagnosis

As discussed earlier, CS cannot be definitively diagnosed by in utero imaging. Low-risk patients with no prior family history of congenital abnormalities do not routinely have additional ultrasonography evaluation past the 20-week detailed scan, thus leading to an inability to detect cases of CS that develop, or become radiographically apparent, during the third trimester. However, a series of findings including family history, risk factors, and concerning prenatal imaging can be strongly suggestive. If a CS syndrome is suspected, further testing via chorionic villus sampling or amniocentesis can be used to identify specific genetic abnormalities. These tests include, but are not limited to, FGFR-1, FGFR-2, FGFR-3, and TWIST-1 gene mutations. Furthermore, CS syndromes may be detected using noninvasive prenatal testing, because CS has become included on certain skeletal dysplasia panels. The advent of full genome sampling has greatly added to the recent knowledge of genetic mutations that cause these conditions.

Prenatal Work-up and Considerations for Delivery

At present, there are no available prenatal treatment options for infants with CS or other cranial anomalies. However, prenatal recognition of possible CS can provide the impetus for further work-up and predelivery counseling. When CS is suspected, the patient should be referred to a tertiary center capable of managing the infant and potential complications during and after birth. A detailed family history should be obtained to identify past cases of CS, syndactyly, heart defects, or any other congenital malformations by a medical geneticist. A thorough ultrasonographic examination and consultation by a perinatologist is necessary, as described earlier. If initial assessment of the heart shows any concerning findings, a fetal echocardiogram should be obtained. The patient should be counseled on the ultrasonography findings and the expected prognosis for developmental outcomes of the infant, and should be given the option of termination, if appropriate.

If suspicion for a syndromic CS exists given the presence of syndactyly or central nervous system or cardiac abnormalities, diagnostic genetic evaluation of the fetus should be offered via chorionic villus sampling or amniocentesis depending on the gestational age of the fetus. Consultation with a medical geneticist is recommended, given the large number of syndromic forms of CS with variable expression and phenotypes. In a large prospective cohort of CS cases, approximately 21% had an identifiable genetic disorder.[42] Although identification of a genetic mutation does not directly affect management, it can play an impactful role in the prenatal and postnatal care of the infant.

Delivery should be conducted at a tertiary care facility, because these infants can develop feeding and breathing difficulties and commonly require a large multidisciplinary team capable of managing their potential challenges and complications. The mode of delivery should be determined based on standard obstetric indications, but, if fetal head circumference is significantly larger than normal, a theoretic increased risk for labor dystocia is present. However, a trial of labor should be considered and cesarean delivery reserved for usual obstetric indications.

Neonates with CS have a higher rate of birth complications relative to neonates with normal skulls.[11,33] This finding includes higher rates of fetal malposition, including abnormal cephalic and breech presentations, with the deflexed position found to be the most common. The noncompliance of the suture also increases rates of trauma as it passes through the narrow birth canal, including postnatal cephalohematomas and maternal perineal lacerations. Unplanned cesarean section in cases of undiagnosed CS seem to be increased (19.7%,[11] 30%[43]). In a study by Weber and colleagues,[33] when CS was diagnosed prenatally, cesarean section was performed more frequently (45%) relative to the normal controls (22%). However, all of the current studies of prenatal diagnosis of CS have been performed retrospectively, which induces significant observer bias when reviewing imaging.

POSTNATAL EVALUATION
History and Physical Examination

CS is most commonly diagnosed after birth, and cranial abnormalities are commonly noted at the time of delivery or shortly after. History should include evaluation for symptoms suggestive of increased ICP (lethargy, vomiting, visual disturbance, or headaches), multiple gestations or abnormal uterine line, family history of CS or associated syndromes, and screening for common risk factors. Focused physical examination should begin with evaluation of the head from above looking down, followed by the front, and then both sides. This method allows physicians to see the head shape, ears, and facial features from many perspectives and improves the ability to detect abnormalities. The head should also be palpated for palpable ridges suggestive of sutural fusion. Measurements of the head should be taken, including circumference, maximal cranial width, and maximal cranial length. Along with visual inspection, a CI can be used to numerically describe the general head shape. This index is calculated by dividing the maximum width by the length.

Neurocognitive evaluation should be performed after birth to evaluate for appropriate or delayed development when concerns arise. The severity of developmental delays can be variable along a spectrum ranging from none to severe even within a specific syndrome. In addition, neonates with syndromic concerns should be evaluated for other associated anomalies. The eyes and orbits should be examined for brow asymmetries, downward slanting of palpebral fissures, hypertelorism or hypotelorism, proptosis, strabismus, and lagophthalmos. A fundoscopic examination should be performed to evaluate for papilledema. The face should also be examined for asymmetries such as deviation of the nasal root, ear anomalies, midface hypoplasia, cleft lip/palate, and deviation of the mandible. The hands and feet should be evaluated for syndactyly or other limb anomalies.

Radiographic Imaging

An accurate differential and probable diagnosis is essential when considering postnatal imaging. Conditions such as cutis aplasia and DP typically do not require radiographic imaging and are managed conservatively without surgery. In contrast, CS and encephalocele both require surgical correction and, as such, preoperative imaging is imperative. When CS is suspected based on examination, radiographic imaging may provide confirmation of suture closure, evaluation of brain or other skull anomalies, and may assist with surgical planning. Plain film radiographs were once routinely used as the initial radiographic screening tool for most cranial anomalies. However, even the best images can be difficult to interpret and, as such, most clinicians use CT imaging as the sole modern gold standard for cranial anomaly assessment. MRI can also be used because this provides optimal visualization of the brain, but it provides less information regarding bony anatomy. This information is important in the case of encephaloceles because the contents of the neural tissue herniating outside the cranial vault require assessment. Selective use of radiographic imaging is imperative because it carries risks. These risks include the frequent need for anesthesia to keep the patient still, as well as the risk of ionizing radiation with CT scan. The amount of radiation that each child is exposed to differs between institutions and CT scanners; however, most centers use a low-dose protocol that minimizes risks without affecting image quality. Concerns have arisen suggesting that there will be a significant increase in soft tissue malignancies as a result of overuse of neonatal CT imaging. However, to date, an increased incidence of soft tissue tumors such as sarcoma has been only theoretic and has not been observed in modern medicine.

APPROACH TO MANAGEMENT
Multidisciplinary Care

Management of neonatal cranial anomalies requires a multidisciplinary team, frequently including pediatrics, plastic surgery, neurosurgery, ophthalmology, radiology, genetics, speech-language pathology, audiology, physical and occupational therapy, psychology, and social work. Initial team evaluation should occur within a few days to weeks of the suspected or confirmed diagnosis. If warranted, surgical correction is often performed within the first year of life; however, it is often delayed until 3 to 9 months of age depending on the anomaly and planned surgical intervention. The reason for the delay is that both neonatal anesthesia and intraoperative blood loss are better tolerated the larger the neonate is at the time of surgery. In addition, cranial bone remains cartilaginous in the initial weeks to months of life, making surgical repairs more difficult until adequate ossification has occurred.

Nonsurgical Interventions

Both DP and cutis aplasia are managed with nonsurgical intervention. DP is managed with a combination of supine repositioning and torticollis stretching exercises. Helmet orthosis is another treatment option and is often reserved for more severe cases because compliance (helmet must be worn 23 h/d for 2–3 months consistently) and expense ($2000–$3000 out of pocket) are concerns with this treatment. Cutis aplasia is typically treated with topical moisturizing dressings that promote epithelization (skin growth) at the scalp vertex for several weeks to months. Even in severe cases in which significant cranial bone is absent at birth, cranial ossification can be completed within the first year of life. Rarely is surgical intervention required until later in life, and this is often simply to remove an area of scalp alopecia that results where the cutis aplasia manifested.

Surgical Interventions

The particular surgical procedure required to address each specific cranial abnormality varies depending on the diagnosis. In general terms, neonatal cranial procedures for CS can be categorized as follows. Strip craniectomy involves the surgical excision of a fused cranial suture and can be done either endoscopically or through an open approach. This technique often requires helmet orthosis to obtain satisfactory head shapes with future compensatory brain growth. Cranial vault remodeling/expansion involves the removal, reshaping, and repositioning of cranial bones and can involve either part (front, side, or back) of the cranial vault or the entire skull (**Fig. 6**). Fronto-orbital advancement is one form or cranial vault remodeling/expansion in which the supraorbital bar and forehead are advanced anteriorly to correct metopic, unicoronal,

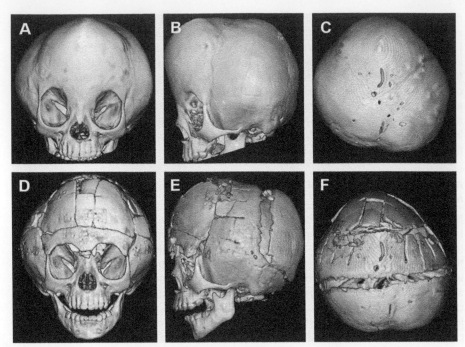

Fig. 6. (*A–C*) Preoperative 3D CT images of a child born with Pfeiffer syndrome and complex multisuture CS. This patient shows cloverleaf or kleeblattschädel head shape. (*D–F*) Postoperative 3D CT scan with improved head shape following multistage surgical reconstruction including posterior cranial vault distraction followed by fronto-orbital advancement.

and bicoronal CS. Encephaloceles are typically treated with surgical removal of the herniating neural tissue, repair of the dural lining, and reconstitution of the cranial vault to prevent further herniation.

Complications

Complications related to neonatal cranial procedures are rare but, when they occur, they can be devastating. Severe complications are most commonly related to anesthesia, intraoperative blood loss, and postoperative infections. Rare occurrences such as cerebral spinal fluid leak, new-onset seizures, and stroke are possible following these procedures. However, even mild complications such as wound infection/dehiscence and hematoma/seroma are rare occurrences and conservative management is often successful at managing these conditions without a return to the operating theater.

SUMMARY

Cranial anomalies are rare but improved imaging techniques are allowing more frequent and accurate identification in utero. Accurate diagnosis is essential for radiographic planning of appropriate treatment strategies. Treatments vary from nonoperative to complex intracranial procedures depending on the specific cranial anomaly. As such, perinatologists remain at the forefront of in utero identification and initial early management.

Best Practices

What is the current practice?

- Routine prenatal imaging should assess for cranial anomalies, including CS, DP, cutis aplasia, and encephaloceles.

- Specific structures to be evaluated include head shape, cranial contour, bony continuity, intracranial structures, facial development, skeletal development, syndactyly, heart, and other vital organs.

- Family history should increase suspicion for a CS involving a syndrome. Findings on prenatal imaging may indicate further investigation with amniocentesis or chorionic villus sampling for common genetic mutations. If a cerebral malformation is suspected, fMRI may be indicated, which can also provide information regarding head shape anomalies.

- Neonates with cranial anomalies should be managed at a tertiary care medical center with high-risk perinatology and neonatologists capable of handling complications during and after delivery.

- There are no current in utero treatments for cranial anomalies.

What changes in current practice are likely to improve outcomes?

- Improvements in prenatal imaging may provide improved and earlier detection of rare cranial anomalies.

- Increased awareness of potential cranial anomalies during routine imaging may increase the rate of prenatal diagnosis.

- Early diagnosis of CS and other cranial anomalies provides the opportunity for genetic testing, prenatal counseling with family, and transfer to a tertiary center with multidisciplinary teams capable of providing optimal care with these complex patients.

- Although few studies have been conducted, there is good evidence that neonates with cranial anomalies have higher rates of complications during and after delivery relative to normal neonates. Early diagnosis of cranial anomalies may decrease rates of complications, although this has not been reported in the literature.
  - Swanson J, Oppenheimer A, Al-Mufarrej F, et al. Maternofetal trauma in craniosynostosis. Plast Reconstr Surg 2015;136(2):214e–22e.
  - Weber B, Schwabegger AH, Oberaigner W, et al. Incidence of perinatal complications in children with premature craniosynostosis. J Perinat Med 2010;38(3):319–25.

Summary statement

- Improved imaging has increased the rate and accuracy of prenatal diagnosis of cranial anomalies. Early diagnosis is essential for optimal management of these complex problems. Perinatologists and neonatologists remain at the forefront of in utero identification and initial early management.

REFERENCES

1. Peitsch WK, Keefer CH, LaBrie RA, et al. Incidence of cranial asymmetry in healthy newborns. Pediatrics 2002;110(6):e72.

2. Helfer TM, Peixoto AB, Tonni G, et al. Craniosynostosis: prenatal diagnosis by 2D/3D ultrasound, magnetic resonance imaging, and computed tomography. Med Ultrason 2016;18(3):378–85.

3. Slater BJ, Lenton KA, Kwan MD, et al. Cranial sutures: a brief review. Plast Reconstr Surg 2008;121(4):170–8.

4. Persing JA, Jane JA, Shaffrey M. Virchow and the pathogenesis of craniosynostosis: a translation of his original work. Plast Reconstr Surg 1989;83(4):738–42.

5. Sgouros S, Goldin JH, Hockley AD, et al. Intracranial volume change in childhood. J Neurosurg 1999;91(4):610–6.

6. Lapeer RJ, Prager RW. Fetal head moulding: finite element analysis of a fetal skull subjected to uterine pressures during the first stage of labour. J Biomech 2001; 34(9):1125–33.

7. Persing JA. Management considerations in the treatment of craniosynostosis. Plast Reconstr Surg 2008;121(1):1–11.

8. Buchanan EP, Xue AS, Hollier LH. Craniosynostosis syndromes. Plast Reconstr Surg 2014;134(1):128e–53e.

9. Roscoili T, Elakis G, Cox TC, et al. Genotype and clinical care correlations in craniosynostosis: findings from a cohort of 630 Australian and New Zealand patients. Am J Med Genet C Semin Med Genet 2013;163C(4):259–70.

10. Shuper A, Merlob P, Grunebaum M, et al. The incidence of isolated craniosynostosis in the newborn infant. Am J Dis Child 1985;139(1):85–6.

11. Swanson J, Oppenheimer A, Al-Mufarrej F, et al. Maternofetal trauma in craniosynostosis. Plast Reconstr Surg 2015;136(2):214e–22e.

12. Selber J, Reid RR, Chike-Obi CJ, et al. The changing epidemiologic spectrum of single-suture synostoses. Plast Reconstr Surg 2008;122(2):527–33.

13. Opperman LA, Sweeney TM, Redmon J, et al. Tissue interactions with underlying dura mater inhibit osseous obliteration of developing cranial sutures. Dev Dyn 1993;198(4):312–22.

14. Roth DA, Bradley JP, Levine JP, et al. Studies in cranial suture biology: Part II. Role of the dura in cranial suture fusion. Plast Reconstr Surg 1996;97(4):693–9.

15. Wilkie AO. Craniosynostosis: genes and mechanisms. Hum Mol Genet 1997; 6(10):1647–56.

16. Thompson DN, Malcolm GP, Jones BM, et al. Intracranial pressure in single-suture craniosynostosis. Pediatr Neurosurg 1995;22(5):235–40.

17. Renier D, Sainte-Rose C, Marchac D, et al. Intracranial pressure in craniostenosis. J Neurosurg 1982;57(3):370–7.

18. Tahiri Y, Bartlett SP, Gilardino MS. Evidence-based medicine: nonsyndromic craniosynostosis. Plast Reconstr Surg 2017;140(1):177e–91e.

19. Speltz ML, Collett BR, Wallace ER, et al. Intellectual and academic functioning of school-aged children with single suture craniosynostosis. Pediatrics 2015;135(3): 615–23.

20. Raybaud C, DiRocco C. Brain malformation in syndromic craniosynostoses, a primary disorder of white matter: a review. Childs Nerv Syst 2007;23(12):1379–88.

21. Fontana SC, Belinger S, Daniels D, et al. Longitudinal assessment of developmental outcomes in infants undergoing late craniosynostosis repair. J Craniofac Surg 2018;29(1):25–8.

22. Kane AA, Mitchell LE, Craven KP, et al. Observations on a recent increase in plagiocephaly without synostosis. Pediatrics 1996;97:877–85.

23. Positioning and sudden infant death syndrome (SIDS): update. American Academy of Pediatrics Task Force on Infant Positioning and SIDS. Pediatrics 1992;89: 1120–6.

24. Mulliken JB, Vander Woude DL, Hansen M, et al. Analysis of posterior plagiocephaly: deformational versus synostotic. Plast Reconstr Surg 1999;103(2):371–80.

25. Argenta LC, David LR, Wilson JA, et al. An increase in infant cranial deformity with supine sleeping position. J Craniofac Surg 1996;98:1216–8.

26. Turk AE, McCarthy JG, Thorne CH, et al. The "back to sleep campaign" and deformational plagiocephaly: is there a cause for concern? J Craniofac Surg 1996;7:12–8.

27. Bruneteau RJ, Mulliken JB. Frontal plagiocephaly: synostotic, compensational, or deformational. Plast Reconstr Surg 1992;89(1):21–31.
28. Littlefield TR, Kelly KM, Pomatto JK, et al. Multiple-birth infants at higher risk for development of deformational plagiocephaly. Pediatrics 1999;103(3):565–9.
29. Huang MH, Gruss JS, Clarren SK, et al. The differential diagnosis of posterior plagiocephaly: true lambdoid synostosis versus positional molding. Plast Reconstr Surg 1996;98(5):765–74.
30. Andrews BT, Meara JG. Reconstruction of frontoethmoidal encephalocele defects. Atlas Oral Maxillofac Surg Clin North Am 2010;18(2):129–38.
31. Cohen MM Jr. Etiopathogenesis of craniosynostosis. Neurosurg Clin North Am 1991;2(3):507–13.
32. Ketwaroo PD, Robson CD, Estroff JA. Prenatal imaging of craniosynostosis syndromes. Semin Ultrasound CT MR 2015;36(6):53–64.
33. Weber B, Schwabegger AH, Oberaigner W, et al. Incidence of perinatal complications in children with premature craniosynostosis. J Perinat Med 2010;38(3):319–25.
34. Fjortoft MI, Sevely A, Boetto S, et al. Prenatal diagnosis of craniosynostosis: value of MR imaging. Neuroradiology 2007;49(6):515–21.
35. Agochukwu NB, Solomon BD, Muenke M. Impacts of genetics on the diagnosis and clinical management of syndromic craniosynostoses. Childs Nerv Syst 2012;28(9):1447–63.
36. Cohen MM Jr, Kreiborg S. New indirect method for estimating the birth prevalence of Apert syndrome. Int J Oral Maxillofac Surg 1992;21(2):107–9.
37. Apert ME. De l'acrocephalosyndactylie. Bull Soc Med Hop Paris 1906;23:1310.
38. Crouzon F. Dysostose cranio-faciale héréditaire. Bull Mem Soc Med Hop Paris 1912;33:545.
39. Pfeiffer RA. Dominant hereditary acrocephalosyndactylia. Z Kinderheilkd 1964;90:301 [in German].
40. Kress W, Schropp C, Lieb G, et al. Saethre-Chotzen syndrome caused by TWIST 1 gene mutations: functional differentiation from Muenke coronal synostosis syndrome. Eur J Hum Genet 2006;14:39.
41. Agochukwu NB, Doherty ES, Muenke M. Muenke syndrome. In: Pagon RA, Bird TD, Dolan CR, et al, editors. GeneReviews. Seattle (WA): University of Washington; 1993. Available at: https://www.ncbi.nlm.nih.gov/books/NBK1415/. Accessed August 22, 2018.
42. Wilkie AO, Byren JC, Hurst JA, et al. Prevalence and complications of single-gene and chromosomal disorders in craniosynostosis. Pediatrics 2010;126:391–400.
43. Heliovaara A, Vuola P, Hukki J, et al. Perinatal features and rate of cesarean section in newborns with nonsyndromic craniosynostosis. Childs Nerv Syst 2016;32(7):1289–92.

Peripartum Management of Neonatal Pierre Robin Sequence

Louis F. Insalaco, MD[a], Andrew R. Scott, MD[b,c,d],*

KEYWORDS

- Pierre Robin sequence • Micrognathia • Glossoptosis • Cleft palate

KEY POINTS

- Pierre Robin sequence (PRS) is a triad of micrognathia, glossoptosis, and cleft palate with varying effects on airway and feeding.
- PRS may occur as an isolated anomaly or in conjunction with additional syndromic features.
- Most patients can be managed safely with nonsurgical measures.
- Surgical options may include tracheostomy, tongue-lip adhesion, or mandibular distraction osteogenesis (MDO).
- MDO is the only surgical option that addresses the underlying cause of the child's airway obstruction and feeding difficulty with long lasting effects.

INTRODUCTION

Pierre Robin sequence (PRS) is a triad of micrognathia, glossoptosis, and U-shaped cleft palate. The earliest descriptions of people with such orofacial malformations can be traced as far back as 1700 BC carved into the ancient clay tablets of Babylon.[1] In recent medical literature, the first report of the combination cleft palate and micrognathia was by Fairbairn[2] in 1846. Similar reports of palate and mandibular anomalies were subsequently made by Lannelongue and Menard[3] in 1891 and Shukowsky[4] in

Financial Disclosures: No conflicts of interest and nothing to disclose.
[a] Department of Otolaryngology–Head and Neck Surgery, Boston Medical Center, 830 Harrison Avenue, First Floor, Boston, MA 02118, USA; [b] Department of Pediatric Otolaryngology, Floating Hospital for Children, Tufts Medical Center, 800 Washington Street, Box 850, Boston, MA 02111, USA; [c] Facial Plastic Surgery, Floating Hospital for Children, Tufts Medical Center, 800 Washington Street, Box 850, Boston, MA 02111, USA; [d] Cleft Lip and Palate Team, Floating Hospital for Children, Tufts Medical Center, 800 Washington Street, Box 850, Boston, MA 02111, USA
* Corresponding author. Tufts Medical Center, 800 Washington Street, Box 850, Boston, MA 02111.
E-mail address: ascott@tuftsmedicalcenter.org

https://doi.org/10.1016/j.clp.2018.07.009
0095-5108/18/© 2018 Elsevier Inc. All rights reserved.
perinatology.theclinics.com

1911. It was not until 1923 and later in 1934 that a full description of the triad of micrognathia, glossoptosis, and cleft palate were described by French stomatologist, Pierre Robin,[5,6] whose name became eternally linked with the condition. Up until the second half of the twentieth century, the term "Pierre-Robin syndrome" was commonly used.[7] This term, although still in limited use today, is actually a misnomer because the condition is the result of a cascade of events that is caused by a single, underlying anomaly, in this case, micrognathia. The more appropriate terminology is to refer to this condition as Pierre Robin sequence or more simply Robin sequence.[8,9] The incidence of this relatively rare disorder is generally accepted to be approximately 1 in 8500,[10] but may vary by race and even geographic location.[11]

CAUSE

Hypoplasia of the mandible, either from a primary growth disturbance or from hyperflexion of the neck, before 9 weeks in utero is thought to be the inciting factor in PRS. Normally the palatal shelves fuse between the 8th and 10th week of gestation. In PRS, the presence of a small jaw results in a posteriorly and superiorly displaced tongue, positioning the tongue between the 2 palatal shelves, thereby preventing their fusion.[11]

Most cases of PRS are isolated cases in nonsyndromic children. The percentage of children that present with PRS as part of a broader syndrome has been reported to be between 25% and 46%.[12,13] A thorough examination and high level of suspicion may point the physician toward a diagnosis of Nager, Stickler, or velocardiofacial syndrome, to name a few. In those cases in which PRS presents with limb abnormalities, microtia, or ocular manifestations, conditions such as Cornelia de Lange, Nagar, or Treacher Collins syndrome might be considered, among others.

DIAGNOSIS
Prenatal Evaluation

Ultrasonography is the current standard for prenatal imaging for both screening and diagnostic purposes. There have been several attempts reported in the literature to standardize fetal mandibular measurements using ultrasound.[14,15] High-resolution ultrasonography has made it possible to diagnose micrognathia as early as the second trimester of pregnancy.[16–18] Based on multiple prior studies, Kaufman and colleagues[19] in 2016 proposed an interesting algorithm for prenatal identification of PRS based on the inferior facial angle and degree of glossoptosis on ultrasound (**Fig. 1**). The presence of cleft palate and polyhydramnios has also been shown to be associated with micrognathia, but the low specificity of these measures makes them less useful in prenatal diagnosis of PRS. The algorithm also incorporates prenatal MRI, which has been shown to be highly accurate in the prenatal diagnosis of micrognathia or PRS (**Fig. 2**).[20] Despite the abundance of measurements and algorithms, the examining physician often diagnoses PRS subjectively. Prenatal recognition is important; there may be certain features that, if recognized, may allow for planned delivery of the neonate in a setting where a difficult airway can be managed.[21] These features have not yet been clearly defined, and current management strategies are based on low levels of evidence gleaned through several reported case series. One of the largest reports published was a retrospective study from 2 institutions examining risk factors for urgent airway intervention within 24 hours of delivery. Although the data presented were only subjected to univariate analysis, prematurity, low birth weight, neurologic abnormalities detected on ultrasound, and the presence of a known syndrome were risk factors for early airway intervention. Other studies

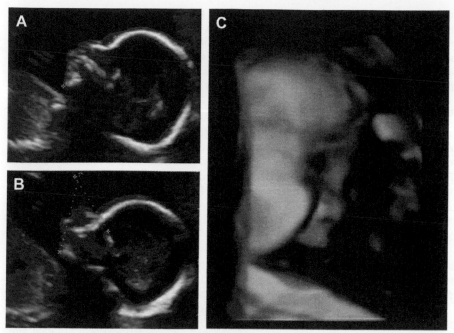

Fig. 1. Prenatal ultrasonography at 24 weeks' gestational age. (*A*, *B*) Calculation of the "jaw index" based on the facial profile. (*C*) Third-trimester 3-dimensional ultrasound reconstruction of a different fetus with PRS.

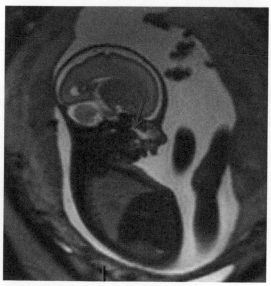

Fig. 2. Third-trimester fetal MRI scan demonstrating a sagittal view of a micrognathic fetus. Note the posterior and superior positioning of the tongue, the tip of which lies in the nasopharynx (*arrow*).

have suggested that polyhydramnios, a finding present in many forms of fetal airway obstruction, should also be considered a risk factor for neonatal airway compromise.[19] It is the senior author's practice to recommend delivery at an institution with pediatric subspecialty airway expertise in those cases of known fetal micrognathia and an additional risk factor outlined above. Management of acute airway obstruction at the time of delivery or later is described later in this article.

Physical Examination

Upon examination of a newborn with PRS, the first feature that is readily noticeable is micrognathia. Micrognathia is characterized by a small, retrusive mandible where the mandibular alveolus is positioned significantly posterior to the maxillary alveolus (**Fig. 3**A). Oral cavity examination reveals a tongue that is forced posteriorly and superiorly due to the shortened mandible length. Palatal examination is notable for a U-shaped cleft palate involving the soft palate and posterior hard palate, sparing the alveolus. The tongue may be positioned within the cleft itself, especially in the supine child (**Fig. 3**B).[11]

Some infants exhibit minimal respiratory symptoms at birth, whereas others have significant airway obstruction, with stertor, retractions, and even cyanosis. These symptoms are usually worse when the child is lying supine, owing to gravity-dependent tongue-base obstruction, which occurs at the level of the oropharynx.[11]

PRS may be the only abnormality noted on newborn examination or may be noted as part of several dysmorphic features owing to a unifying, syndromic diagnosis. For this reason, some children with PRS are robust and vigorous, whereas others may have significant hypotonia (due to underlying neurologic impairment) or worrisome cyanosis (due to structural heart disease, for example). Examination of the ears, eyes, heart, and extremities may point toward a syndromic diagnosis. For this reason, a full evaluation by a geneticist is helpful for categorizing infants with PRS into those with isolated findings and those with additional syndromic features. Given the high rate of Stickler syndrome among infants with PRS, ophthalmology consultation is also recommended as an essential part of the routine workup for a newborn with PRS (**Fig. 4**). In addition, children with neurologic impairment are at a higher risk than their peers with isolated PRS for requiring surgical intervention for airway distress.[22,23]

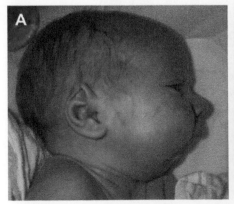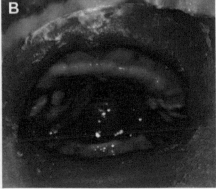

Fig. 3. Glossoptosis and cleft palate in the context of micrognathia (isolated PRS). (*A*) Micrognathia is evident on facial profile. (*B*) The tongue is positioned lying within the cleft palate, filling the space between the lateral palatal shelves.

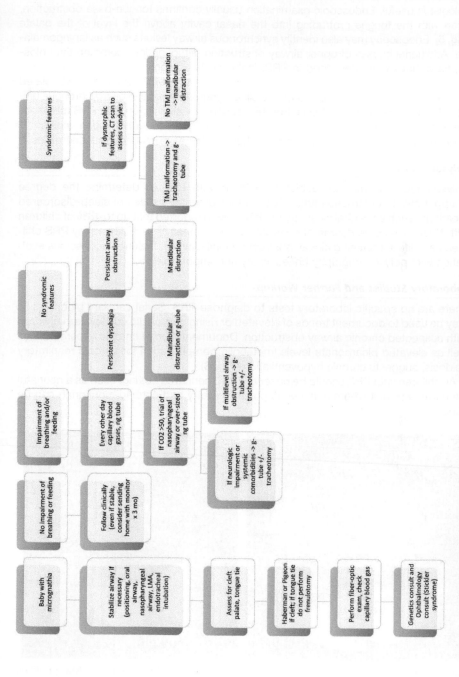

Fig. 4. The senior author's algorithm for managing newborns with PRS. CT, computed tomography; g-tube, surgical gastrostomy tube; mo, months; ng tube, nasogastric feeding tube; TMJ, temporomandibular joint.

Endoscopic Examination

Evaluation of the airway obstruction with fiber-optic nasal laryngoscopy by an otolaryngologist is useful. Endoscopic examination usually confirms tongue-base obstruction, often with the tongue protruding into the nasal cavity above the level of the palate (**Fig. 5**). Endoscopy may also identify synchronous airway lesions such as laryngomalacia. Additional causes of upper airway obstruction, although less common than glossoptosis, have been described in PRS, including lateral pharyngeal wall motion and pharyngeal narrowing without glossoptosis. Some children with syndromic PRS related to craniofacial microsomia or Treacher Collins syndrome may exhibit synchronous unilateral or bilateral choanal atresia. For this reason, not all children with PRS are effectively managed with interventions that target tongue-base obstruction alone.[11,24] Endoscopy as an intubation aid has been shown to increase intubation success rates.[25]

Polysomnography

Polysomnography may be useful in children with PRS to determine the degree of upper airway obstruction and rule out other potential causes of sleep-disordered breathing, such as central sleep apnea. It has been reported that up to 46% of children with PRS have some degree of obstructive sleep apnea.[26] In reality, many PRS children have life-threatening airway obstruction while *awake*, making unconscious evaluation with polysomnography unnecessary and impossible.[11]

Laboratory Studies and Further Workup

There are no specific laboratory tests to diagnose PRS. Serial capillary blood gases may be used to document trends of elevated or rising carbon dioxide levels in children with suspected chronic airway obstruction. Documentation of chronic hypercarbia as well as elevated bicarbonate levels (metabolic compensation for chronic respiratory acidosis) suggests chronic hypoventilation (**Fig. 6**).

All children with PRS should be observed in a monitored setting, such as a neonatal intensive care unit where continuous pulse oximetry and cardiac monitoring can be used.[11]

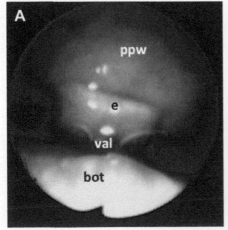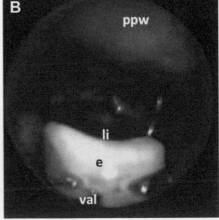

Fig. 5. Endoscopic views of neonatal tongue base airway obstruction. (*A*) Marginalized airway in supine position at rest. (*B*) With crying and agitation, the tongue moves forward and the caliber of the pharyngeal airway improves. bot, base of tongue; e, epiglottis; li, laryngeal inlet; ppw, posterior pharyngeal wall; val, vallecula.

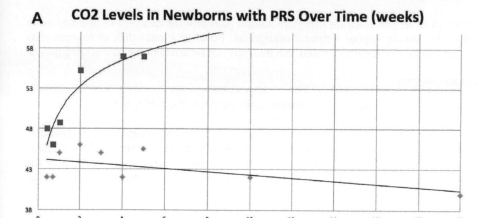

A **CO_2 Levels in Newborns with PRS Over Time (weeks)**

- ◆ PRS not requiring intervention (mean for 5 patients)
- ■ PRS requiring surgical intervention (mean for 6 patients)
- —Log. (PRS requiring surgical intervention (mean for 6 patients))
- —Linear (PRS not requiring intervention (mean for 5 patients))

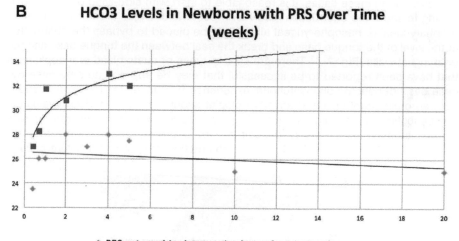

B **HCO_3 Levels in Newborns with PRS Over Time (weeks)**

- ◆ PRS not requiring intervention (mean for 5 patients)
- ■ PRS requiring surgical intervention (mean for 6 patients)
- —Linear (PRS not requiring intervention (mean for 5 patients))
- —Log. (PRS requiring surgical intervention (mean for 6 patients))

Fig. 6. Serial capillary blood gas measurements may provide an objective measure of chronic hypoventilation in infants. Laboratory values collected during the neonatal period and early infancy in newborns with PRS. Red: those infants who required surgical intervention; green: those infants who did not require airway surgery. (*A*) Carbon dioxide levels in capillary blood. (*B*) Bicarbonate levels in capillary blood.

Failure to thrive in children with PRS is the result of decreased caloric intake and increased work of breathing. Monitoring weight gain in these children is important to determine the need for further intervention. PRS children will typically lose weight in the first week of life as most infants do, but failure to return to birth weight by day of life 14 or to demonstrate minimum weight gain of 4 ounces (~115 g) every week thereafter should trigger further investigation. Fortified breast milk or formula may be used to increase caloric intake, but this may not be sustainable as the child grows.

MANAGEMENT

PRS is not an all or none phenomenon, and, as such, there is a wide variation in the degree of intervention necessary to manage this condition. The clinician caring for these patients may not be trained in the execution of all of the following techniques, but should be aware of resources that exist for the management of this condition. Ultimately, it is important that the neonatologist have a firm understanding of the appropriate consultants to notify in order to provide optimal care for these children with complex airway and feeding needs.

Initial Airway Management

Upon initial evaluation of the micrognathic child, a determination is made based on history and physical examination of the degree, if any, of respiratory distress that the child is in. Airway symptoms in PRS may vary from no distress, to apneas, increased accessory muscle use, failure to thrive, cyanosis, and ultimately, respiratory insufficiency.[27] With no signs of respiratory distress, the best intervention may be no intervention. Nevertheless, many children do display signs of respiratory distress, and in these cases, it is reasonable to start with side-lying or prone positioning to see if the obstruction resolves. If postural changes are not effective, an oropharyngeal or nasopharyngeal airway can be placed to bypass the obstruction at the level of the tongue base and break the seal between the tongue base and the pharyngeal walls (**Fig. 7**).[11] There are several types of customized oral appliances that have been reported to be successful that may be appropriate on a case-by-case basis depending on institutional experience.[28–30] In severe cases of obstruction, an otolaryngologist and anesthesiologist should be consulted for evaluation for intubation as an option, including fiber-optic intubation. In rare cases, when intubation is extremely difficult or not possible, tracheostomy may be required. In most cases of PRS, if acute obstruction or respiratory failure occurs,

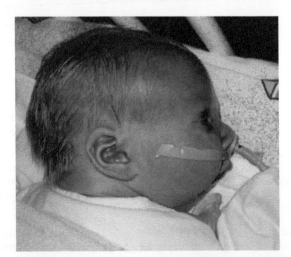

Fig. 7. A nasopharyngeal airway (nasal trumpet) provides an intermediate step between simple repositioning and a more invasive surgical intervention.

the airway can be stabilized with placement of a laryngeal mask airway (LMA). Even among those newborns in whom direct laryngoscopy is not possible, an LMA will stabilize the airway so long as there is no syngnathia (fusion of the upper and lower jaw) or severe ankylosis prohibiting jaw opening.[21]

Feeding Considerations

There is a direct synergy between breathing and feeding in infants. Infants with a normal oropharynx and larynx are able to breathe and feed simultaneously, owing to the cephalad positioning of the infantile larynx as compared with the adult larynx and the interdigitation of the uvula and soft palate with the epiglottis. With this in mind, it should come as no surprise that many patients with PRS are unable to effectively feed orally as a result of the posteriorly displaced tongue base and presence of cleft palate. Such anatomic impairments may result in inadequate oral intake and ultimately failure to thrive. It is important to understand that in the PRS population, failure to thrive is the result of 2 mechanisms: decreased caloric intake and increased work of breathing.

The degree of feeding difficulty in PRS children is highly variable. Assessing the degree of feeding difficulty should be done over the course of at least 1 to 2 weeks in order to establish a trend in feeding difficulties and weight gain before determining the most appropriate intervention. Consultation with an experienced feeding therapist is important in determining the degree of feeding difficulty and the appropriate strategies and interventions required to facilitate growth.

Initial strategies that may be implemented in PRS infants are the same as those for any child with cleft palate. Mothers should be instructed to avoid breast feeding because the child will be unable to maintain an adequate suckle. Delivery of breast milk or formula with a specialized bottle such as the Haberman or Pigeon Feeders should be used instead.

Children with more severe feeding difficulty require supplemental nutrition via nasogastric or orogastric catheter. If prolonged or unsuccessful attempts at nasogastric feeding are encountered, surgical intervention should be considered. Correction of the underlying micrognathia through neonatal mandibular distraction osteogenesis (MDO) will reliably improve failure to thrive in children with isolated PRS.[31] The details of this procedure will be discussed later. Alternatively, surgical gastrostomy tube (g-tube) placement may be performed to provide a more secure and manageable source of enteral nutrition. Gastrostomy tube placement carries with it the associated risks of neonatal abdominal surgery including general anesthesia, infection, dislodgement, abdominal adhesions, scarring, and prolonged oral aversion.[32]

Nonsurgical Management

Nonsurgical management options for children with PRS may include positioning changes, nasopharyngeal airway placement, and/or enteral nutritional support. Retrospective reviews have suggested that most children with PRS can be successfully managed nonoperatively.[13,22,33–35] Caouette-Laberge and colleagues[34] assigned children with PRS into 3 separate groups based on the severity of their respiratory and feeding symptoms and found the likelihood of surgical intervention to be much more likely in the children with the most severe symptoms. A recent review by Albino and colleagues[36] suggests that children with consistent weight gain and mild to moderate obstructive sleep apnea on polysomnography with a mean apnea/hypopnea index (AHI) <20 events/h may be managed with conservative measures until symptoms of upper airway obstruction eventually improve later in childhood. However, it should be noted that in infants and children an AHI of 10 or greater is considered severe sleep apnea. Therefore, it is the authors' strong belief that when chronic, severe upper airway obstruction is documented in infancy, some form of intervention is mandated.

For most infants with PRS who are discharged home with positioning strategies or airway appliances alone, it is the senior author's practice to provide these families with an outpatient respiratory monitoring system. As infants mature, positional and appliance-based modes of intervention may be weaned, with the ultimate goal of discontinuation.[37,38]

Surgical Management

Many children with PRS are unable to tolerate oropharyngeal stents and nasopharyngeal airways, and management of these devices may overwhelm both providers and parents alike. In these children, as well as children with severe airway obstruction and feeding difficulties, surgical intervention is appropriate. Despite the obvious need for surgical intervention in many cases, there are no widely accepted guidelines or treatment algorithms.

Tongue-lip adhesion

Shukowsky[4] in 1911 recognized PRS as a serious condition in which the neonate developed congenital stridor with cyanosis that he attributed to rearward displacement of the tongue. His solution to this problem was to advance the tongue forward by suturing the tongue to the lower lip. This description was the first description of what remains a commonly used surgical technique, the tongue-lip adhesion (TLA).

There are several different approaches to TLA, the modern iteration of which also tethers the base of tongue anteriorly to the mandible (**Fig. 8**).[39] A TLA is typically maintained throughout the first year of life and is taken down at the time of cleft palate repair, around 1 year of age. A recent meta-analysis showed an average of 50% reduction in OSA in PRS children.[40] The success rate of this procedure in preventing further airway intervention has been reported to be as high as 89%.[41]

Despite its proven success, TLA disrupts physiologic swallowing function, exacerbating the child's dysphagia, assuring the need for enteral nutritional support via

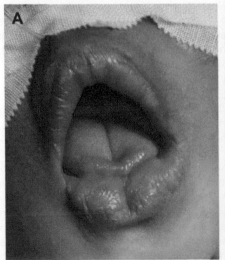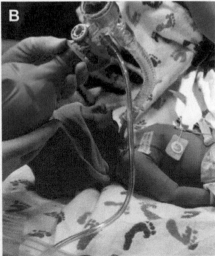

Fig. 8. Surgical airway interventions for tongue base obstruction associated with micrognathia. (A) Tongue lip adhesion. (B) Tracheotomy.

nasogastric or gastrostomy tube in the weeks following the procedure and in many cases throughout infancy.[13,33,41] The results of TLA have also been less than encouraging with a recent study by Resnick and colleagues[42] showing only a 50% rate of resolution of OSA in PRS patients. As a result, most institutions have abandoned this procedure, with only about 26% of surgeons endorsing its use in a recent survey.[43]

Tracheotomy

Traditionally, tracheotomy was reserved for patients who failed TLA. A tracheotomy is the definitive management for upper airway obstruction, and in PRS, it effectively bypasses obstruction at the level of the base of tongue. Despite its effectiveness, tracheotomy in children has potential long-term morbidity and mortality. Complications include sudden airway obstruction from accidental decannulation or mucous plugging, bleeding, wound care issues, tracheal stenosis, and speech and swallowing impairment.[44] Furthermore, managing a tracheotomy in a child has significant emotional, financial, and physical impact on family caregivers.[45] Although tracheotomy is certainly a valuable tool in the management of severe PRS, only 16% of surgeons surveyed use this method regularly.[43] However, in some children with neurologic impairment, lung disease, or those with multilevel airway obstruction or additional mandibular anomalies, tracheotomy remains the only efficacious treatment option (**Fig. 9**).

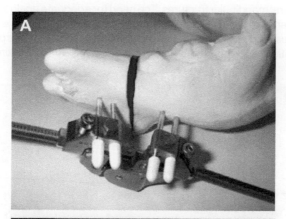

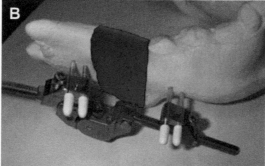

Fig. 9. The concept behind MDO. A medical model with external multivector distractor demonstrates of how lengthening regenerate bone (*red*) results in improved mandibular projection over time. (*A*) Formation of regenerate following initial mandibulotomy. (*B*) Formation of regenerate bone following gradual linear distraction.

Mandibular distraction osteogenesis

MDO has gained popularity among craniofacial surgeons because it offers definitive management of PRS in the neonatal period. The technique involves creating osteotomies, either freehand or through the use of preoperative virtual surgical planning, in the mandible with placement of external or internal distraction hardware that allows for slow anterior advancement of the mandible at a pace that allows for creation of new bone as well as gradual expansion of the associated soft tissues (**Fig. 10**). The earliest form of MDO involved hardware in the form of pins that were secured to the mandible and protruded through the skin overlying the jaw. An external device or distractor was secured to the pins, allowing for mobilization of the mandibular segments.

More recently, buried or internal distraction devices have become increasingly popular. Such devices obviate an external hardware component and result in reduced external scarring compared with external distractors. Drawbacks of this technique include more extensive operative dissection, greater potential for developing open bite deformity (especially with the use of unidirectional, linear distractors), and the need for a more invasive second procedure to remove the hardware, which places the facial nerve at risk (**Fig. 11**).[11]

Only those children with severe upper airway obstruction are candidates for neonatal MDO. It is the authors' opinion that even those children who did not require intubation preoperatively cannot be safely extubated immediately following surgery, when the airway is *worse*. Following mandibular distraction, one should expect significant pain owing to the presence of bilateral mandibular fractures. The need for adequate analgesia coupled with postoperative edema and volume shifts makes the postoperative airways of these infants even more tenuous than their preoperative state. It is the senior author's practice to leave neonatal distraction patients intubated and sedated for approximately 5 days

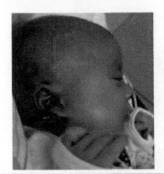
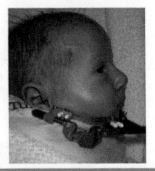

Buried Univector Device		External Multivector Device	
Advantages	*Disadvantages*	*Advantages*	*Disadvantages*
Less exposed hardware, greater stability	Unable to inspect hardware	Easy to inspect hardware	Less stable
Less facial scarring	Univector distraction, potential asymmetry and/or open bite	Multivector distraction, immediate correction of asymmetry and/or open bite	Facial scars
Easier care during consolidation	Additional surgery for removal	Simple procedure for removal	More care required during consolidation
	CT for precise vector planning	No imaging required in most cases	
	More expensive	Less expensive	

Fig. 10. Side-by-side comparison of the benefits and limitations of buried univector versus external multivector neonatal MDO.

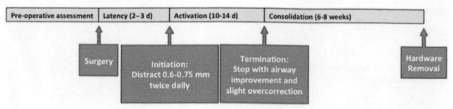

| Pre-operative assessment | Latency (2–3 d) | Activation (10-14 d) | Consolidation (6-8 weeks) |

Surgery

Initiation: Distract 0.6-0.75 mm twice daily

Termination: Stop with airway improvement and slight overcorrection

Hardware Removal

Fig. 11. Timeline of neonatal MDO favored by the authors.

postoperatively. Those requiring intubation before surgery are typically extubated on postoperative days 6 to 7. Distraction typically begins 36 to 48 hours postoperatively, and a distraction rate of 1.0 to 1.5 mm per day is implemented. At this rate, the airway caliber is adequately improved by postoperative day 5, at which point analgesic requirements have diminished and postoperative edema has improved. Distraction is continued until the appropriate position of the mandible is reached. The hardware is left in place for approximately 6 weeks in what is known as a consolidation period, where bone mineralization occurs, strengthening the mandible (**Figs. 12–15**). Depending on whether an external or buried system is used, the hardware is subsequently removed in the office without the need for general anesthetic or in the operating room. Risks of neonatal MDO include facial scarring, facial nerve injury, hardware malfunction, and risk of injury to tooth buds or the inferior alveolar nerves.[32]

Patient selection
Proper patient selection is paramount in effecting good outcomes. Rogers and colleagues[41] suggested several characteristics that may identify those children with the highest likelihood of failing TLA with the GILLS score. The GILLS score stands

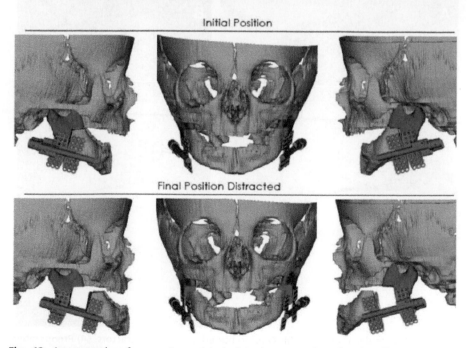

Initial Position

Final Position Distracted

Fig. 12. An example of computer-assisted virtual surgery for planning linear/univector neonatal mandibular distraction.

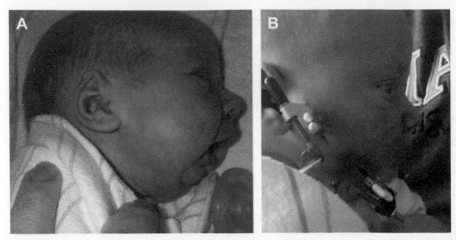

Fig. 13. Initial results of neonatal MDO. (*A*) Preoperative mandibular profile. (*B*) Mandibular profile at completion of activation phase using external multivector distraction system (note the slight overprojection).

for Gastroesophegeal reflux, *I*ntubation preoperatively, *L*ate operation (>2 weeks of age), *L*ow birth weight (<2.5 kg, 5.5 lbs), and *S*yndromic diagnosis. Each of these 5 characteristics is assigned one point, and a score of greater than 3 points suggests a failure rate of greater than 40%. A 2015 study by Flores and colleagues[46] looked at variable predictive failure of mandibular distraction and found that children with

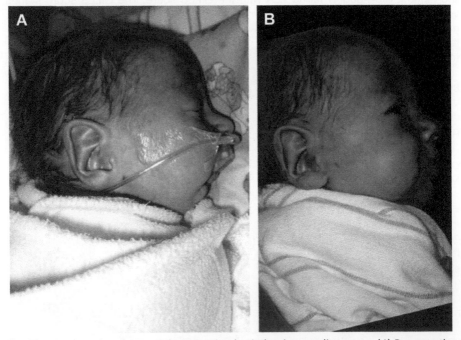

Fig. 14. Initial results of neonatal MDO using buried univector distractors. (*A*) Preoperative mandibular profile. (*B*) Mandibular profile at completion of activation phase. The photographs are 12 days apart.

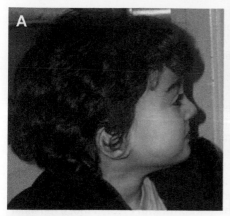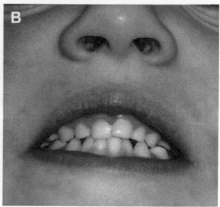

Fig. 15. Long-term results following neonatal MDO for failure to thrive and airway obstruction. (*A*) Facial scarring and maintained mandibular projection 6 years following surgery using external multivector system. (*B*) Occlusion at 4 years of age (similar patient).

gastroesophageal reflux, age greater than 30 days, neurologic anomaly, airway anomalies other than laryngomalacia, intact palate, and preoperative intubation were at highest risk of failure, defined as postprocedure tracheostomy, limited improvement in AHI, or death by apnea. It is clear from these 2 studies that some of the same attributes predictive of failure with TLA are predictive of failure with MDO and that otherwise healthy children with PRS are most likely to have a favorable outcome with either TLA or MDO. There are exceptions to this trend, such as children with Stickler syndrome, who have been shown to fare equally as well as their peers with surgical intervention.[32,47] For this reason, it is the authors' opinion that it is the presence of neurologic impairment and/or additional levels of airway obstruction that limit the potential efficacy of MDO in infants with PRS, and alternative treatment options, such as tracheotomy and/or tongue lip adhesion, should be considered.

Given the fact that concomitant airway anomalies and gastroesophageal reflux are negative predictors of success of MDO, it has been proposed by some groups to evaluate for these preoperatively with 24-hour pH probe, imaging, and/or direct laryngoscopy/bronchoscopy. Such diagnostic procedures may help the surgeon identify patients better managed with a tracheotomy versus MDO.[31,48]

Outcomes

MDO has been shown to have more favorable outcomes than TLA with multiple sources reporting decreased rates of tracheotomy and gastrostomy tube placement.[49–52] MDO has also been shown to have an advantage over TLA with regards to improvement in obstructive sleep apnea. A prospective study by Khansa and colleagues[53] in 2017 compared MDO, TLA, and conservative management of PRS. It showed that those in the MDO group had the greatest reduction in AHI compared with TLA or conservative management. No significant difference was seen between the 3 groups in this study in days to extubation or discharge, change in weight percentile, requirement of gastrostomy tube, or residual obstructive sleep apnea. Other studies examining the rate of gastrostomy tube placement in high-volume TLA centers versus high-volume MDO centers suggest that g-tube insertion is more common among TLA patients compared with MDO patients.[11]

Ultimately, favorable outcomes will be dependent on selecting the most appropriate intervention for the child depending on their symptoms, examination findings, and comorbidities. For this reason, it is of extreme importance to have a care team familiar with and experienced with all treatment options. The care team and family must be aware of the success rates and limitations of the proposed interventions so that expectations are set appropriately before instituting a certain treatment plan.

SUMMARY

PRS is a relatively rare condition seen in neonates and results in variable degrees of airway obstruction, feeding difficulty, and failure to thrive. A thorough workup by a specialized team familiar with the management of this condition is necessary before instituting any type of treatment. Treatment options vary considerably depending on the severity of the condition. Conservative treatment options are often attempted first and include prone positioning, airway appliances, and enteral nutrition. Such conservative measures can be expected to adequately address hypoventilation and feeding impairment in up to 60% of newborns with PRS. In those remaining children that fail conservative therapy, surgical options include TLA, MDO, and tracheotomy. The success of these approaches, especially TLA or MDO, is often contingent on the neurologic status of the child, with those who are neurologically impaired being more likely to require tracheotomy and gastrostomy tube placement. MDO is a newer technique that has been shown to have more favorable outcomes than TLA and is currently the most common surgical intervention used for PRS. With proper evaluation and care, most children with isolated PRS can go on to live full and healthy lives.

Best Practices

What is the current practice?

Pierre Robin Sequence (PRS)
- Initial diagnosis based on presence of micrognathia, glossoptosis, and cleft palate with varying degrees of airway obstruction and feeding difficulty
- Most PRS children can be managed with observation and nonsurgical measures
- In more severe cases, surgical intervention with tracheotomy, tongue-lip adhesion (TLA), or mandibular distraction osteogenesis (MDO) should be considered

What changes in current practice are likely to improve outcomes?

- The recent shift toward performing MDO over TLA in PRS patients has been shown to decrease rates of tracheostomy tube and gastrostomy tube placement.

Major Recommendations
- Management of upper airway obstruction in children with PRS is best approached conservatively with nonoperative measures attempted first if possible

Rating for the Strength of the Evidence
- C: Recommendation based on consensus, usual practice, expert opinion, disease-oriented evidence, and case series for studies of diagnosis, treatment, prevention, or screening

Bibliographic Sources
- See References

Summary Statement

PRS is a rare condition with varying degrees of severity that may cause airway obstruction, feeding difficulties, or failure to thrive. Management options are considered on an individual basis based on clinical evaluation by qualified specialists who may judge the severity of the child's symptoms. In most cases, nonsurgical management is adequate. In cases where surgical management is indicated, MDO should be considered a first-line treatment over TLA or tracheostomy alone.

REFERENCES

1. Poswillo D. The aetiology and surgery of cleft palate with micrognathia. London: Hunterian Lecture delivered at the Royal College of Surgeons; 1968.
2. Fairbairn P. Mth. J Med Sci 1846;6:280.
3. Lannelongue OM, Menard V. Affections congenitales. Paris: Asselin et Houzeau; 1891.
4. Shukowsky, W. P. Jb. Kinderheilk 1911;73:459.
5. Robin P. La chute de la base de la langue considerée comme une nouvelle cause de gene dans la respiration nasopharyngienne. Bull Acad Med (Paris) 1923;89: 37–41.
6. Robin P. Glossoptosis due to atresia and hypotrophy of the mandible. Am J Dis Child 1934;48:541.
7. Randall P, Krogman WM, Jahina S. Pierre Robin and the syndrome that bears his name. Cleft Palate J 1965;2:237–46.
8. Shprintzen RJ. The implications of the diagnosis of Robin sequence. Cleft Palate Craniofac J 1992;29:205–9.
9. Breugem CC, Courtemanche DJ. Robin sequence: clearing nosologic confusion. Cleft Palate Craniofac J 2010;47(2):197–200.
10. Bush PG, Williams AJ. Incidence of robin anomalad (pierre robin syndrome). Br J Plast Surg 1983;36:434.
11. Scott AR, Tibesar RJ, Sidman JD. Pierre Robin Sequence: evaluation, management, indications for surgery, and pitfalls. Otolaryngol Clin North Am 2012;45: 695–710.
12. Pasyayan HM, Lewis MB. Clinical experience with the Robin sequence. Cleft Palate J 1984;21(4):270–6.
13. Evans AK, Rahbar R, Rogers GF, et al. Robin sequence: a retrospective review of 115 patients. Int J Pediatr Otorhinolaryngol 2006;70:973–80.
14. Malas MA, Ungor B, Tagil SM, et al. Determination of dimensions and angles of mandible in the fetal period. Surg Radiol Anat 2006;28(4):364–71.
15. Captier G, Faure JM, Baumler M, et al. Prenatal assessment of the anteroposterior jaw relationship in human fetuses: from anatomical to ultrasound cephalometric analysis. Cleft Palate Craniofac J 2011;48(4):465–72.
16. Lee W, McNie B, Chaiworapongsa T, et al. Three-dimensional ultrasonographic presentation of micrognathia. J Ultrasound Med 2002;21:775–81.
17. Rotten D, Levaillant JM, Martinez H, et al. The fetal mandible: a 2D and 3D sonographic approach to the diagnosis of retrognathia and micrognathia. Ultrasound Obstet Gynecol 2002;19:122–30.
18. Bronshtein M, Blazer S, Zalel Y, et al. Ultrasonographic diagnosis of glossoptosis in fetuses with Pierre Robin sequence in early and mid pregnancy. Am J Obstet Gynecol 2005;193(4):1561–4.
19. Kaufman MG, Cassady CI, Hyman CH, et al. Prenatal identification of pierre robin sequence: a review of the literature and look towards the future. Fetal Diagn Ther 2016;39(2):81–9.
20. Resnick CM, Kooiman TD, Calabrese CE, et al. An algorithm for predicting Robin sequence from fetal MRI. Prenat Diagn 2018;38(5):357–64.
21. Tonsager SC, Mader NS, Sidman JD, et al. Determining risk factors for early airway intervention in newborns with micrognathia. Laryngoscope 2012; 122(Suppl 4):S103–4.
22. Meyer AC, Lidsky ME, Sampson DE, et al. Airway interventions in children with Pierre Robin Sequence. Otolaryngol Head Neck Surg 2008;138(6):782–7.

23. Handley SC, Mader NS, Sidman JD, et al. Predicting surgical intervention for airway obstruction in micrognathic infants. Otolaryngol Head Neck Surg 2013; 148(5):847–51.

24. Sher AE. Mechanisms of airway obstruction in Robin sequence: implications for treatment. Cleft Palate Craniofac J 1992;29(3):224–31.

25. Manica D, Schweiger C, Sekine L, et al. The role of flexible fiberoptic laryngoscopy in Robin Sequence: a systematic review. J Craniomaxillofac Surg 2017; 45(2):210–5.

26. Khayat A, Bin-Hassan S, Al-Saleh S. Polysomnographic findings in infants with Pierre Robin sequence. Ann Thorac Med 2017;12(1):25–9.

27. van Lieshout MJ, Joosten KF, Mathijssen IM, et al. Non-surgical and surgical interventions for airway obstruction in children with Robin Sequence. J Craniomaxillofac Surg 2016;44(12):1871–9.

28. Pielou WD, Allen A. The use of an obturator in the management of the Pierre Robin syndrome. Dent Pract Dent Rec 1968;18(5):169–72.

29. Oktay H, Baydas B, Ersöz M. Using a modified nutrition plate for early intervention in a newborn infant with Pierre Robin sequence: a case report. Cleft Palate Craniofac J 2006;43(3):370–3.

30. Bacher M, Sautermeister J, Urschitz MS, et al. An oral appliance with velar extension for treatment of obstructive sleep apnea in infants with Pierre Robin sequence. Cleft Palate Craniofac J 2011;48(3):331–6.

31. Mandell DL, Yellon RF, Bradley JP, et al. Mandibular distraction for micrognathia and sever upper airway obstruction. Arch Otolaryngol Head Neck Surg 2004; 130(3):344–8.

32. Goudy SL, Tollefson TT. Complete cleft care: cleft and velopharyngeal insufficiency treatment in children. New York: Thieme; 2015. p. 21–36.

33. Kirschner RE, Low DW, Randall P, et al. Surgical airway management in Pierre Robin sequence: is there a role for tongue-lip adhesion? Cleft Palate Craniofac J 2003;40(1):13–8.

34. Caouette-Laberge L, Bayet B, Larocque Y. The Pierre Robin sequence: review of 125 cases and evolution of treatment modalities. Plast Reconstr Surg 1994;93: 934–42.

35. Tomaski SM, Zalzal GH, Saal HM. Airway obstruction in the Pierre Robin sequence. Laryngoscope 1995;105:111–4.

36. Albino FP, Wood BC, Han KD, et al. Clinical factors associated with the non-operative airway management of patients with robin sequence. Arch Plast Surg 2016;43(6):506–11.

37. Lander TA, Scott AR. Mandibular distraction. Chapter in: Complete cleft care: cleft and velopharyngeal insufficiency treatment in children. New York: Thieme; 2015.

38. Parhizkar N, Saltzman B, Grote K, et al. Nasopharyngeal airway for management of airway obstruction in infants with micrognathia. Cleft Palate Craniofac J 2011; 48(4):478–82.

39. Argamaso RV. Glossopexy for upper airway obstruction in Robin sequence. Cleft Palate Craniofac J 1992;29:232–8.

40. Camacho M, Noller MW, Zaghi S, et al. Tongue lip adhesion and tongue repositioning for obstructive sleep apnoea in Pierre Robin Sequence: a systematic review and meta-analysis. J Laryngol Otol 2017;131(5):378–83.

41. Rogers GF, Murthy AS, LaBrie RA, et al. The GILLS score: part I. Patient selection for tongue-lip adhesion in Robin sequence. Plast Reconstr Surg 2011;128(1): 243–51.

42. Resnick CM, Dentino K, Katz E, et al. Effectiveness of tongue-lip adhesion for obstructive sleep apnea in infants with robin sequence measured by polysomnography. Cleft Palate Craniofac J 2016;53(5):584–8.
43. Collins B, Powitzky R, Robledo C, et al. Airway management in pierre robin sequence: patterns of practice. Cleft Palate Craniofac J 2014;51(3):283–9.
44. D'Souza JN, Levi JR, Park D, et al. Complications following pediatric tracheotomy. JAMA Otolaryngol Head Neck Surg 2016;142(5):484–8.
45. Hartnick CJ, Bissell C, Parsons SK. The impact of pediatric tracheotomy on parental caregiver burden and health status. Arch Otolaryngol Head Neck Surg 2003;129(10):1065–9.
46. Flores RL, Greathouse ST, Costa M, et al. Defining failure and its predictors in mandibular distraction for Robin sequence. J Craniomaxillofac Surg 2015; 43(8):1614–9.
47. Mingo K, Lander TA, Sampson DE, et al. Use of external distraction devices eliminates the need for preoperative computed tomography in infants with isolated Pierre Robin sequence. JAMA Facial Plast Surg 2016;18(2):95–100.
48. Andrews BT, Fan KL, Roostaeian J, et al. Incidence of concomitant airway anomalies when using the University of California, Los Angeles, protocol for neonatal mandibular distraction. Plast Reconstr Surg 2013;131(5):1116–23.
49. Tibesar RJ, Scott AR, McNamara C, et al. Distraction osteogenesis of the mandible for airway obstruction in children: long-term results. Otolaryngol Head Neck Surg 2010;143(1):90–6.
50. Lidsky ME, Lander TA, Sidman JD. Resolving feeding difficulties with early airway intervention in Pierre Robin Sequence. Laryngoscope 2008;118:120–3.
51. Scott AR, Tibesar RJ, Lander TA, et al. Mandibular distraction osteogenesis in infants younger than 3 months. Arch Facial Plast Surg 2011;13(3):173–9.
52. McCarthy JG, Schreiber J, Karp N, et al. Lengthening the human mandible by gradual distraction. Plast Reconstr Surg 1992;89:1.
53. Khansa I, Hall C, Madhoun LL, et al. Airway and feeding outcomes of mandibular distraction, tongue-lip adhesion, and conservative management in pierre robin sequence: a prospective study. Plast Reconstr Surg 2017;139(4):975e–83e.

Vascular Anomalies

Adam B. Johnson, MD, PhD[a],*, Gresham T. Richter, MD[b]

KEYWORDS

- Vascular anomalies • Hemangioma • Lymphatic malformation

KEY POINTS

- Vascular anomalies are congenital lesions of abnormal vascular development broadly divided, using the International Society for the Study of Vascular Anomalies classification scheme, into malformations and tumors, of which the infantile hemangioma is most common.
- Unless function is affected, vascular anomalies rarely need treatment during the neonatal period.
- Beard-like distributed segmental infantile hemangiomas should trigger vigilant observation of the airway for subglottic disease.
- Large cervicofacial lymphatic malformations can cause congenital high airway obstructive syndrome (CHAOS) and require intubation or a surgical airway at birth.
- Lymphatic malformations can be treated with sclerotherapy and/or surgery, depending on resources, skillset, and extent of the lesion.

INTRODUCTION
Hemangiomas

A hemangioma is a benign vascular tumor that consists of a collection of hyperplastic proliferative endothelial cells arterioles. They can be divided into infantile hemangiomas (IHs), rapidly involuting congenital hemangiomas (RICHs), and noninvoluting congenital hemangiomas (NICHs) (**Box 1**).

IHs are the most common hemangiomas and tumors of infancy (**Fig. 1**). They occur in approximately 5% to 10% of children.[1] Nearly 60% of these lesions occur in the head and neck.[2] They are not usually present at birth but appear anywhere from a few days to 3 weeks postnatal life. They rapidly enlarge over a short span of time and will enter a quiescent period as early as 6 months of age. Rapid growth can lead to ulceration, disfigurement, or obstruction of vital structures. After the child is a year old, the lesion will begin to shrink and involute, and bulky lesions can leave

[a] Otolaryngology–Head and Neck Surgery, University of Arkansas for Medical Sciences, 1 Children's Way Slot 836, Little Rock, AR 72201, USA; [b] Otolaryngology–Head and Neck Surgery, University of Arkansas for Medical Sciences, 1 Children's Way, Slot 836, Little Rock, AR 72201, USA
* Corresponding author.
E-mail address: AJohnson4@uams.edu

Clin Perinatol 45 (2018) 737–749
https://doi.org/10.1016/j.clp.2018.07.010
0095-5108/18/Published by Elsevier Inc.

Box 1
International Society for the Study of Vascular Anomalies classification system (abbreviated for the scope of this article)

Vascular tumors

Hemangiomas
 Infantile
 Noninvoluting congenital
 Rapidly involuting congenital

Kasposiform Hemangioendothelioma

Vascular malformations

Slow-flow
  CM
  VM
  LM

Fast-flow
  Arterio-VM

---

behind a fibro-fatty residuum. Ultrasound and MRI can be helpful in the diagnosis of deep lesions with evidence of arteriole and venous channels in a globular vascular mass. Ultrasound of these tumors will demonstrate a high-flow vascular lesion with multiple flow voids within the tumor. If history, appearance, and imaging are inconclusive, a biopsy can be performed to histologically demonstrate glucose transporter-1–positive proliferating immature endothelial cells and confirm the diagnosis. The involution of IHs is rarely quick and may require years of patience before they resolve. Multiple studies have shown the differentiation of hemangioma into fibro-fatty tissue; however, the mechanism behind this is still poorly understood.

Treatment of IH in the neonatal period is seldom necessary but may be required during the proliferative period to prevent impending functional or aesthetic complications. Inconspicuous IHs on the body can be simply observed if they do not ulcerate or encroach on vitals areas (ie, vision, airway). Treatment of ulcerative or bleeding hemangiomas may require topical therapy using either silver impregnated creams, topical timolol 0.5%,[3] or flash-lamp pulsed-dye laser for promotion of reepithelization.[4] These treatments can be performed on an outpatient basis.

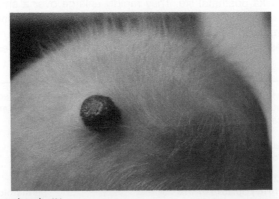

Fig. 1. Pedunculated scalp IH.

Treatment is necessary when an IH has the potential cause major deformity (**Fig. 2**) or compromise function in the airway or orbit. Currently, the treatment of choice is propranolol. When younger than 2 months of age, the patient is treated with a 1 mg/kg dose split 3 times daily, then increased to 2 mg/kg split 3 times daily.[5] Some studies also state that a 3 mg/kg dose can be used. It is recommended that an electrocardiogram be obtained and evaluated by a cardiologist before starting propranolol treatment. The authors' recent work suggests that this may not be necessary with children who are otherwise healthy. In children with a cardiac history, an electrocardiogram should not be avoided and may need to be augmented with an echocardiogram. Surgical treatment may be required in IHs that are pedunculated or have vertical boarders because these are likely to leave residuum. Surgery for these particular lesions can be performed at any time. In fact, the authors recommend that surgery be postponed until the patient is at least 6 months old and when the family is ready for removal. As with any procedure correcting a deformity, these should be removed by age 4 to 5 years old to prevent the child from unwanted attention by their peers.

Segmental facial IHs have a 50% to 60% risk of having associated airway hemangiomas. It is important to solicit if stridor is present in the patient's history and to have a low threshold for use of flexible laryngoscopy. A scope in the clinic setting is useful but evaluation under anesthesia with rigid microlaryngoscopy and bronchoscopy is recommended because this will inform diagnosis and treatment. Segmental airway IH often includes the supraglottis and subglottis. Rarely are supraglottic lesions obstructive. However, when subglottic IHs are encountered, the amount of the airway involved dictates the treatment. For small lesions, an intralesional injection with a steroid mixture of triamcinolone acetonide (40 mg/ml) and betamethasone (6 mg/mL) will expedite shrinking the IH when combined with systemic propranolol therapy.[6] Unresponsive lesions might require laser or open resection. Carbon dioxide laser ablation of subglottic IH has recently fallen out of favor secondary to the increased risk of laryngeal stenosis (5%–25%).[6,7]

Congenital hemangiomas

Congenital hemangiomas are present and at their maximal size on delivery. Sometimes these are confused with other more dangerous vascular tumors or malformations. Congenital hemangiomas are further divided into RICHs and NICHs. Both are Glut-1-receptor–negative; however, RICHs, as the name implies, are present at birth

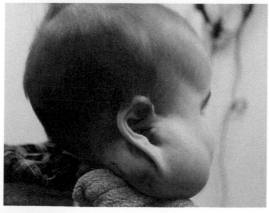

Fig. 2. Large deep parotid IH.

but involute quickly by age 6 to 14 months.[8] Imaging characteristics such as visible vessels and calcifications can help distinguish them from IHs.[9] Seldom is treatment needed except for when they are large and leave behind a fatty residuum. Occasionally, RICHs have an associated risk of hematologic abnormalities such as Kasabach-Merritt phenomenon (KMP) (see later discussion).

NICHs present at birth and grow in proportion with the patient.[9] These lesions generally need to be removed for cure. Vascular staining of the skin from a RICH or a NICH sometimes responds to flash-lamp pulsed-dye or gentle neodymium-doped yttrium aluminium garnet (Nd:YAG) laser therapy. When trying to distinguish between RICH and NICH, it is best to wait until the child is 1 year of age to see if the lesion will rapidly involute. Propranolol is ineffective on these lesions.

LYMPHATIC MALFORMATIONS

Lymphatic malformations (LMs) are slow-flow vascular malformations that are usually present at birth but not always noticed until later in life. These lesions grow by vascular expansion and can be problematic, especially if they become infected and expand rapidly. LMs are arbitrarily categorized based on the size of the predominant cysts within the lesions. Macrocystic (>2 cm), microcystic (<2 cm), or mixed lesions exist. Typically, a contrasted MRI is used to stage and delineate the extent of disease and to determine macrocystic versus microcystic components in involved areas that may not be seen on physical examination. Macrocysts tend to expand next to, and compress, adjacent tissue, whereas microcystic lesions are infiltrative. LMs of the head and neck are further described by their location and prognosis using the de Serres classification scheme. This classification scheme categorizes disease severity based on location and prognosis.[9]

Macrocystic lesions are generally noticed at birth and are commonly found as cervicofacial LMs (**Fig. 3**). These lesions are large and can cause concern for airway problems. Patients with large cervicofacial lesions also have a distinct laryngeal phenotype even without direct airway involvement. Effective treatment of macrocystic LM with surgical resection and sclerotherapy has been demonstrated.[10]

Microcystic LMs can be difficult to treat. They have a high recurrence rate because they infiltrate normal soft tissue with mucosal and skin involvement. Generally, these require excision or interstitial sclerotherapy. Bleomycin sclerotherapy has proven very

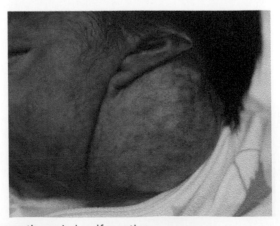

Fig. 3. Large macrocystic cervical malformation.

effective in the treatment of microcystic LM with repeated therapy at 3-month intervals for best results. Risk of pulmonary fibrosis is low but should be discussed with family during each treatment. Doses should be limited to less than 100 units per square meter of body surface area. Carbon dioxide laser and coblation therapy are effective for superficial mucosal vesicular disease. Most LMs are of a mixed architecture, including venous channels, and are named based on the dominant component. Treatment is targeted to the cyst type. Many patients with mixed disease are currently treated with the mechanistic target of rapamycin (mTOR) inhibitor, sirolimus (Rapamune, Rapamycin), with mixed results. Best outcomes from sirolimus seem to result when treatment is initiated in the early neonatal period. However, the length of treatment required is still unclear.

Evidence suggests that macrocystic and microcystic LMs differ in gene expression and growth patterns. Occasionally, LMs will expand secondary to intracystic bleeding or infection in or near the lesion. This rapid growth can change the treatment algorithm at any time. In the neonatal period, LMs can obstruct the airway, causing congenital high airway obstruction syndrome (CHAOS) at birth. CHAOS is usually discovered prepartum via ultrasound and might require an ex utero intrapartum treatment (EXIT) procedure to secure the airway. Fetal MRI is helpful in predicting airway compromise (**Fig. 4**). A surgical airway team should be present for any delivery in which there is question of compromise. Securing the airway might require tracheostomy, especially in de Serre type 5 lesions. The primary goal of treatment then becomes to decannulate the patient as soon as possible through multimodal therapy. The authors' goal is to decannulate the patient within a year of life through multimodal treatment, although this is not always feasible.

VENOUS MALFORMATIONS

Venous malformations (VMs) are slow-flow lesions that are present at birth and composed of a network of serpiginous interconnected veins. They consist of ectatic venous channels that are deficient in vascular smooth muscle and believed to be caused by a defect in a tyrosine kinase pathway. VMs are generally sporadic with a few inheritable forms. They are often mistaken for deep his due their bluish cutaneous hue; however, they have distinct clinical characteristics that help distinguish between them. Unlike IHs, VMs are slow growing, low-flow, and increase in size with elevations in vascular pressure from Valsalva maneuvers, dependency, exercise, or agitation. In

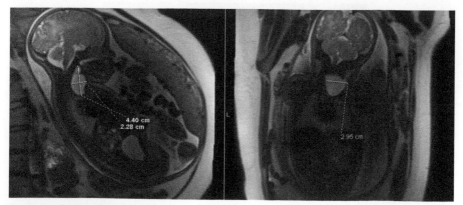

Fig. 4. Fetal MRI of a macrocystic cervical facial LM.

infants, crying will increase the dimension and volume of VMs, making them easier to distinguish. Most VMs are compressible on palpation but may contain small calcifications called phleboliths that occur as the result of prolonged intravascular coagulation. Elevated D-dimers and low fibrinogen may be present in these patients.

In the head and neck, a diagnosis of VM is made easier by placing the malformation in a dependent position to see if the lesion acutely enlarges. The aerodigestive tract is often involved in newborns with head and neck VM, with evidence of blue mucosal staining of compressible lesions (**Fig. 5**). In the neonatal period, these lesions rarely need intervention; however, diagnosis can be confirmed by ultrasound or MRI if necessary (**Fig. 6**). If they do need intervention, superficial lesions of the mucosa and skin can be treated with Nd:YAG (1064 nm wavelength) and gentle Nd:YAG laser therapy, respectively. Focal lesions can be treated with sclerotherapy, such as bleomycin, and/or excision. Excision of a large lesion can be preoperatively embolized with N-butyl cyanoacrylate (glue) to reduce bleeding and simplify removal by better delineating their borders. Treatment of a VM is generally reserved for at least 6 months of age. Sirolimus has also been incorporated into the treatment of complex VMs, with evidence of decreased disease burden and pain, with improvement of coagulation abnormalities.

KAPOSIFORM HEMANGIOENDOTHELIOMAS

Kaposiform hemangioendotheliomas (KHEs) are extremely rare lesions that occur in the neonatal period. They are generally large, greater than 5 cm, and have an incidence of 0.071 per 100,000 and, therefore, consensus on management of these lesions is not concise. These lesions are aggressive vascular tumors that can complicated by platelet trapping causing thrombocytopenia. This trapping secondary to KHEs is known as KMP. KHEs are complicated by KMP more than 70% of the time.[11] This can be a life-threatening complication. KHEs are generally treated with hematological agents such as vincristine, steroids, or sirolimus. These systemic medications can aid with resolution of KMP when it occurs with KHE, as well as resolve the KHE. Surgical treatment of these lesion is rarely warranted. If the lesion is small and can be removed in full without much consequence, then early intervention is indicated.

CAPILLARY MALFORMATIONS

Capillary malformations (CMs) are commonly discovered in the neonatal period and should not be confused with IHs. CMs will present with a well-delineated vascular

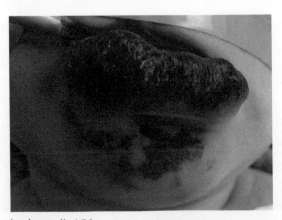

Fig. 5. Large complex lower lip VM.

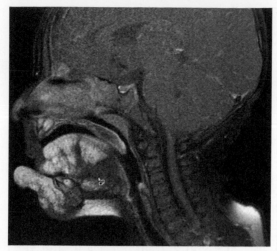

Fig. 6. MRI of a complex lower lip and tongue VM.

stain but, unlike IHs, vertical growth will not occur during the neonatal period or thereafter. They will alternate in color base and increase the infant's temperature, blood pressure, and activity. CMs are also described as port-wine stains. Patients with CMs that involve the trigeminal nerve (V) distribution should be examined for Sturge-Weber syndrome, a condition that describes a patient with a CM and associated meningeal involvement, glaucoma, and/or developmental delays. This is very rare, even in patients with cranial nerve V1 CMs. CMs can be treated with laser therapy superficially to alleviate the disease, with the rare likelihood of cure. Flash-lamp pulsed-dye and alexandrite lasers have been used in the treatment of CMs. Topical sirolimus has also proven beneficial to augment laser therapy results (**Table 1**).

SURGICAL TECHNIQUE

Hemangiomas (IH, RICH, NICH)
1. Incision should be planned to parallel relaxed skin tension lines if possible.
2. Local anesthetic plus hemostatic agents, such as epinephrine, should be injected.
3. The skin incision is carried down to the subcutaneous fat on the lower incision first so as not obstruct the surgeon's view with bleeding.
4. Mostly blunt dissection should occur in the subcutaneous plan, leaving fat on muscle.
5. The upper incision should connect to the subcutaneous plane to allow for removal of the entire lesion.
6. Any residual hemangioma can treated with bipolar cautery.
7. Small flap should be raised on either side of the incision.
8. The wound is closed under minimal tension.
9. Flash-lamp pulsed-dye laser therapy is appropriate for any residual vascular staining.

LMs (large macrocystic lesions)
1. Incision should be planned to parallel relaxed skin tension lines if possible.
2. Local anesthetic plus hemostatic agents, such as epinephrine, should be injected.

Table 1
Indications or contraindications

Lesion	Observation	Medical	Injection or Sclerotherapy	Laser	Surgical
IH	Lesions of the trunk and extremities	Large lesions in critical areas, airway lesions	Airway lesions	Vascular stain and ulcerated bleeding lesions	Small lesions in noncritical cosmetic areas
RICH	All lesions	None	None	Residual vascular stain	Only for residuum, if present
NICH	None	None	None	Residual vascular stain	Required later in life
LM	Rare	Lesions in critical areas	Large macrocystic lesion, with contraindications for surgical treatment		Small focal lesion and part of multimodal therapy
VM	Rare	None	Aid for excision or lesions that cannot be excised; For unresectable lesions	Superficial lesions, multimodal therapy	Cure for focal lesions, part of multimodal therapy for complex
Arterio-VM	None	For unresectable lesions	Multimodal therapy	Multimodal therapy	
KHE	None	For all lesions	None	None	Biopsy for diagnosis
CM	Some	Topical	None	All, as desired	

3. Nerve monitoring is indicated near larger named nerves, such as the facial nerve.
4. Careful dissection using mostly blunt dissection should be carried out around the lesion circumferentially, the goal is not to enter the lesion.
5. Often, the disruption of the sac happens after 270° of dissection. Although not ideal, this allows the surgeon to easily remove the final portion of the lesion.
6. Any unresectable LM should be sclerosed before wound closure under direct visualization.
7. A drain without suction along with a pressure dressing should be applied for a week to reduce persistent drainage and seroma formation.

VM (possible)

1. VMs usually require general anesthesia.
2. Presurgical planning is most important, orientation of incisions should be within the relaxed skin tension lines when possible but must allow access to the lesion.
   a. All preoperative imaging should be available before and during the case.
3. Nerve monitoring is imperative when dealing with a lesion near cranial nerve VII (this can be done with active visualization or electronic nerve monitor).
4. Any large vessel feeders should be dissected early but ligated last.
   a. Early ligation of large vessels will cause engorgement and create more difficulty with the dissection.
5. Bleeding during the procedure should be controlled with bipolar (nonstick) cautery.
   a. If bleeding near a nerve ensues, gelfoam-soaked thrombin is helpful in gaining hemostasis.
6. Sclerotherapy (bleomycin) can be performed after the lesion is resected.
7. Drain placement should account for the large amount of dead space.
8. Closure should consist of standard cosmetic closures, use of flaps and grafts should be implemented for wounds under tension.
9. Gentle Nd:YAG laser therapy can be used for early treatment of superficial skin VM or later treatment of residual superficial disease after resection.

Postoperative care

- Patients with large or critical excisions should be admitted.
- If a drain was placed
  - Most drains can some out the day before discharge.
  - LMs should have a drain in place for at least a week secondary to these lesions to form seromas.
- Steroids should be used in lymphatic and VMs.

OUTCOMES

Excision of a hemangioma is generally a cure for the disease. Propranolol (low-dose beta-blocker therapy) is a useful adjunct in IHs to keep the lesions small for a smaller scar and better cosmetic outcome. Observation of flat lesions in inconspicuous areas allows for good outcomes and minimal to no irregularities in the skin. RICHs only require resection of the residuum but that should be delayed a year to allow for maximal regression. Smaller lesions will resolve rapidly on their own. NICHs will not resolve on their own and will eventually need resection, which is generally a cure.

Macrocystic LMs treated with sclerotherapy before resection are more difficult to remove. Although sclerotherapy as a single modality has been shown to be effective, in the author's experience, resection is more definitive and the scar is minimal. Sclerotherapy is reserved for patients with disease that cannot be removed owing to risk of damage to critical structures.

Medical management of problematic IHs (those that pose risk to function and form) with beta-blocker therapy is more than 90% effective in reducing the burden of disease. Surgical excision, laser therapy, and intralesional steroid injections are also used in select IH as an adjunct or alternative to propranolol.

Vascular malformations rarely require urgent therapy during the neonatal period. Mixed, large, or complex vascular malformations are best managed with multidisciplinary service geared toward multimodal and staged interventions that include medical therapy (sirolimus), surgical resection, and intralesional therapy (sclerotherapy).

Major recommendations

- Use the ISSVA classification scheme for diagnosis of neonatal vascular anomalies.

- Begin with propranolol (beta-blocker) therapy for problematic IHs.

- Subglottic (airway) hemangiomas need to be explored in patients with a beard-like distribution segmental IH.

- Congenital hemangiomas should be observed, if possible, for the first year to see if they will rapidly involute (RICH) or not involute at all (NICH).

- Isolated macrocystic lesions can be treated with early surgical resection or sclerotherapy for best results.

- Sirolimus medical therapy should be considered early for mixed, massive, and high de Serres stage LMs.

- VMs are infiltrative and require selective therapy with Nd:YAG laser, sclerotherapy, or surgical resection with preoperative glue embolization.

- KHE requires early diagnosis and medical management to improve life-threatening thrombocytopenia.

REFERENCES

1. Kilcline C, Frieden IJ. Infantile hemangiomas: how common are they? A systematic review of the medical literature. Pediatr Dermatol 2008;25(2):168–73.
2. Huoh KC, Rosbe KW. Infantile hemangiomas of the head and neck. Pediatr Clin North Am 2013;60(4):937–49.
3. Chang CS, Kang GC. Efficacious healing of ulcerated infantile hemangiomas using topical timolol. Plast Reconstr Surg Glob Open 2016;4(2):e621.
4. Li Y, Hu Y, Li H, et al. Successful treatment of ulcerated hemangiomas with a dual-wavelength 595- and 1064-nm laser system. J Dermatolog Treat 2016;27(6):562–7.
5. Drolet BA, Frommelt PC, Chamlin SL, et al. Initiation and use of propranolol for infantile hemangioma: report of a consensus conference. Pediatrics 2013;131(1):128–40.
6. Darrow DH. Management of infantile hemangiomas of the airway. Otolaryngol Clin North Am 2018;51(1):133–46.
7. Cotton RT, Tewfik TL. Laryngeal stenosis following carbon dioxide laser in subglottic hemangioma. Report of three cases. Ann Otol Rhinol Laryngol 1985;94(5 Pt 1):494–7.
8. Mulliken JB, Enjolras O. Congenital hemangiomas and infantile hemangioma: missing links. J Am Acad Dermatol 2004;50(6):875–82.
9. Gorincour G, Kokta V, Rypens F, et al. Imaging characteristics of two subtypes of congenital hemangiomas: rapidly involuting congenital hemangiomas and non-involuting congenital hemangiomas. Pediatr Radiol 2005;35(12):1178–85.

10. de Serres LM, Sie KC, Richardson MA. Lymphatic malformations of the head and neck. A proposal for staging. Arch Otolaryngol Head Neck Surg 1995;121(5): 577–82.

11. Croteau SE, Liang MG, Kozakewich HP, et al. Kaposiform hemangioendothelioma: atypical features and risks of Kasabach-Merritt phenomenon in 107 referrals. J Pediatr 2013;162(1):142–7.

12. Zhang G, Chen H, Gao Y, et al. Sirolimus for treatment of Kaposiform hemangioendothelioma with Kasabach-Merritt phenomenon: a retrospective cohort study. Br J Dermatol 2018;178(5):1213–4.

13. Chiu YE, Drolet BA, Blei F, et al. Variable response to propranolol treatment of kaposiform hemangioendothelioma, tufted angioma, and Kasabach-Merritt phenomenon. Pediatr Blood Cancer 2012;59(5):934–8.

14. Ji Y, Chen S, Xiang B, et al. Sirolimus for the treatment of progressive kaposiform hemangioendothelioma: a multicenter retrospective study. Int J Cancer 2017; 141(4):848–55.

Choanal Atresia and Other Neonatal Nasal Anomalies

Roy Rajan, MD[a],*, David Eric Tunkel, MD[b]

KEYWORDS

- Congenital nasal anomalies/deformities • Choanal atresia
- Pyriform aperture stenosis • Encephaloceles • Gliomas • Dermoids
- Nasolacrimal duct cysts • Neonatal nasal septal deviations

KEY POINTS

- Congenital nasal deformities can lead to respiratory distress in infancy due to infant preference for nasal breathing and usually need early intervention.
- Choanal atresia is usually treated through a transnasal endoscopic approach and may or may not need stenting; pyriform aperture stenosis can be observed, but severe cases may require sublabial drilling as well as intranasal surgery.
- The evaluation of an infant with suspected encephalocele, glioma, or dermoid may require imaging with both computed tomography and MRI.
- Ophthalmology evaluation and assessment are helpful in nasolacrimal duct cysts.
- Early intervention in significant neonatal nasal septal deformity allows successful correction of nasal airway obstruction.

INTRODUCTION: NATURE OF THE PROBLEM

Although infants are anatomically capable of breathing orally, they are usually considered obligate nasal breathers.[1] Congenital nasal masses and anomalies can cause obstruction, which results in respiratory distress in newborns and infants. These respiratory difficulties often occur with the first attempt at oral feeding. The presence or suspicion of a congenital nasal anomaly is a common reason for urgent consultation with an otolaryngologist. When a catheter cannot be passed through the nasal cavity into the pharynx, choanal atresia or pyriform aperture stenosis should be considered. Occasionally, the examiner will note abnormal nasal contour with or without associated facial anomalies. A nasal mass may be seen externally, near the nasal dorsum, or intranasally on additional examination. In this article, the authors discuss some of

Disclosure Statement: None.
[a] Department of Surgery, Lehigh Valley Health Network, 1210 South Cedar Crest Boulevard, Suite 1100, Allentown, PA 18103, USA; [b] Department of Otolaryngology–Head and Neck Surgery, Johns Hopkins School of Medicine, 601 North Caroline Street, Room 6161B, Baltimore, MD 21287, USA
* Corresponding author.
E-mail address: royrajan@yahoo.com

well. Although transpalatal and transseptal approaches have been used in the past, the overwhelming majority of repairs are now performed transnasally using endoscopes to visualize the atresia plate. "Cold" surgical tools, powered drills/microdebriders, and lasers are used to remove soft tissue and bone. A recent Cochrane review found no randomized trials to help recommend any particular surgical approach, so only the results of case series and clinical experience are left to inform the authors' surgical plans.[4]

The goals of the surgery are to (1) create as large of a choanal opening that anatomic limits allow, usually by removing the atresia plate, resecting the posterior vomer, and drilling the medial bony processes of the medial pterygoids; (2) reline as much of the raw surface of the opened choana with mucosal flaps if possible (**Fig. 3**). Recent reports using mucosal flaps secured by tissue glue seem promising.[5] The choanal resection is principally viewed transnasally with 0° telescopes, but supplemental views of the choana "retrograde" through the nasopharynx can be achieved with angled telescopes or mirrors.

The need for indwelling postoperative stents has been debated, and a recent TRIO Best Practice monograph recommended against the routine use of stents to avoid complications of stenting such as alar injury or infection.[6] The senior investigator does use indwelling stents after the repair of choanal atresia in newborns when the atresia plate is predominantly bony and resection leaves extensive raw surfaces. The authors use a silicone rubber (Silastic) 5 mm tubing in newborns, wrapped around the posterior septum, secured with a suture in a sublabial pocket around the nasal spine (**Fig. 4**). The stents sit well inside the nasal cavity to prevent both alar irritation and the noxious appearance of stents protruding from the nose. One recent series reported the use of multiple mucosal flaps secured with fibrin glue to line resected areas and avoid the need for stents.[5] With or without stent use, parents should be counseled that long-term success of choanal atresia repair may require revision surgeries for removal of granulation, inspection of the choana, and dilation.

Complications/Management

As mentioned earlier, there is an inherent risk of restenosis with choanal atresia and multiple operations may be needed. Diligent follow-up, debridement, and use of antibiotic drops and topical steroids are often used to minimize the need for reoperation

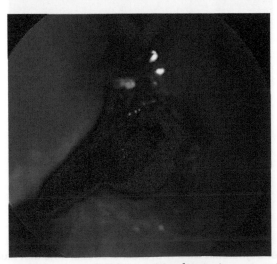

Fig. 3. Choanal atresia plate resected with resection of posterior septum (endoscopic view).

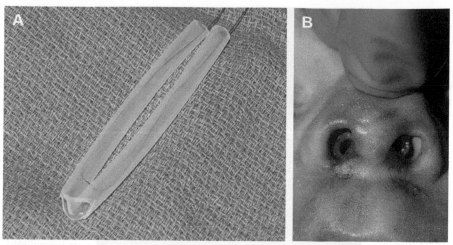

Fig. 4. (*A*) Silastic tubing used to stent after choanal atresia repair, designed to wrap around the back of the septum. (*B*) Stents sit inside the nasal cavity to allow suctioning and avoid alar trauma.

on the atresia/stenosis. The stents, if placed, may cause local infection (dacryocystitis) as well as nasal alar injury, so close follow-up is important.

Postoperative Care

With or without stenting, postoperative care usually consists of nasal saline, suctioning, and use of antibiotic/steroid drops to prevent granulation and minimizing restenosis. Stents are usually removed after 5 to 21 days, although this varies widely among surgeons.[7] Repeat endoscopy is usually necessary for evaluation of the choana, with debridement of granulation and dilation.

Summary/Discussion

Fiberoptic nasal endoscopy and noncontrast axial CT scan are keys to diagnosis, with bilateral choanal atresia likely clinically evident earlier than unilateral disease. A transnasal endoscopic surgical technique is most commonly used, and stenting may or may not be necessary. Close follow-up and care will lead to better results. A workup for syndromic diagnosis such as CHARGE should be performed in infants diagnosed with choanal atresia.

CONGENITAL NASAL PYRIFORM APERTURE STENOSIS

Congenital nasal pyriform aperture stenosis (CNPAS) is an uncommon cause of neonatal nasal airway obstruction where the nasal processes of the maxilla are abnormally prominent causing obstruction in the anterior nasal cavity (**Fig. 5**). Brown first reported a series of infants with CNPAS in 1989, and an association of CNPAS with a central single maxillary mega-incisor (**Fig. 6**) and with craniofacial/central nervous system anomalies such as holoprosencephaly is now well recognized.[8]

Anatomy

The pyriform aperture is the most anterior bony segment of the nasal cavity, formed by the nasal bones superiorly, the nasal processes of the maxilla laterally, and the horizontal maxillary processes inferiorly. The prominence of the medial nasal processes

A comprehensive neurologic and endocrinologic workup should be considered given the associated known comorbidities.

MIDLINE NASAL MASSES

The most common midline nasal masses seen in infancy include dermoids, encephaloceles, and gliomas. Encephaloceles and gliomas are related in that they are derived from defects in the skull base allowing tissue that would normally be intracranial into the nasal cavity (**Fig. 7**). Nasal dermoids also are a result of a defect in development of the anterior neuropore but contain ectodermal and mesodermal derivatives. Other midline nasal masses include tumors, hemangiomas, teratomas, and vascular malformations but will not be discussed in this article. Imaging should always precede biopsy of midline nasal masses in infants, given concerns for bleeding and even more for cerebrospinal fluid (CSF) leak should the masses have an intracranial communication.

An encephalocele is a herniation of cranial contents through a defect in the skull base, and there is usually a communication of CSF with the extracranial mass. Encephaloceles are further characterized by their contents and location of the defect. When only the meninges are herniated, it is considered a meningocele. When brain and meninges are included in the herniated mass, it is called a meningoencephalocele. The incidence of encephaloceles and neural tube defects is declining with the emphasis on prenatal folic acid consumption in expectant mothers.[15] Most babies with anterior encephaloceles are now born in regions underserved by medical care.

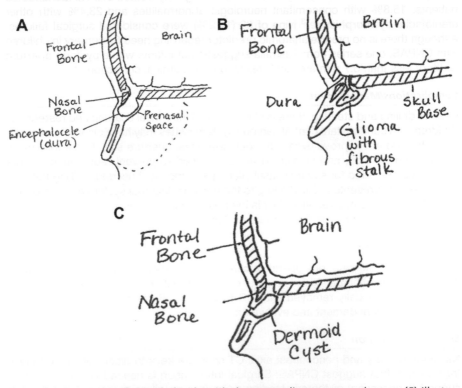

Fig. 7. (A) Illustration of encephalocele with dura extending to prenasal space. (B) Illustration of glioma with a stalk that extends intracranially. (C) Illustration of dermoid cyst in prenasal space extending the skin surface through a tract.

In North America and Europe, the incidence is estimated to be 1 in 30,000 to 40,000 live births, whereas the incidence is as high as 1:5000 to 6000 in Asian populations.[16] Encephaloceles occur usually sporadically, but there is an increased tendency to occur when other neural tube defects and other central nervous system abnormalities are reported in family members.

Gliomas consist of glial tissue that no longer communicates with the CSF-containing subarachnoid space. Five to twenty percent of these lesions have some fibrous stalk that extends intracranially. They do not have familial inheritance and occur more in men (3:2).[17] A nasal dermoid is a cyst that includes skin appendages usually in the prenasal space due to failure of regression of embryonic neuroectoderm. There is usually a sinus tract and associated cyst wall containing epithelium, sebaceous tissue, and/or hair. These lesions can also extend intracranially, with the potential for meningitis or other central nervous system symptoms with enlargement or infection.[18] Dermoid cysts and sinuses are the most common congenital midline nasal mass with an incidence of 1:20,000 to 40,000.[19] Most cases are sporadic with a slight male preponderance.[17] They are usually isolated lesions without other masses or deformities.

Anatomy

Normally, dura projects in utero through the foramen cecum, an anterior skull base opening. By around the seventh week of development, the nasal and frontal bones form from neurocranial tissue, and this dura may extend inferior and posterior to the frontal and nasal bones and anterior to the nasal cartilages to fill the prenasal space.[16,17] When this dura and the neurocranial tissue fail to regress as they normally do, an encephalocele, glioma, or dermoid may result. Hoving's work implicates a failure of closure of the neuropore, causing persistent communication between the brain and skin surface.[20]

Sincipital (anterior), occipital, and basal are the location-based classifications of encephaloceles. Most of the encephaloceles in North America and Europe are occipital encephaloceles, but these occur outside the nasal cavity and will not be further discussed. Sincipital encephaloceles account for 20% of encephaloceles. Basal encephaloceles are even less common and arise more posteriorly between the cribriform plate and superior orbital fissure or posterior clinoid fissure. These present as intranasal masses.

Gliomas present as extranasal (60%), intranasal (30%), or combined lesions (10%).[21,22] Extranasal lesions are smooth, firm, and noncompressible masses that are most commonly seen at the glabella but can be seen down to the nasal tip. Intranasal gliomas are pale masses that may protrude from the nostril. The nasal cavity may be obstructed due to these lesions. Intranasal gliomas most commonly arise from the lateral nasal wall near the middle turbinate and occasionally from the septum.[21,22] Nasal dermoids usually present with a midline dorsal nasal dimple with or without drainage, swelling, or hair growth (**Fig. 8**).

Diagnosis

Scincipital encephaloceles will classically present as a bluish, pulsatile, compressible lesion in the glabella or dorsum of the nose. They will transilluminate and tend to expand when crying, straining, or compressing the jugular veins. Basal lesions may not be as obvious at an early age as they will be intranasal and may not cause initial obstruction. Because there is no connection with the CSF spaces, gliomas do not change in size and do not transilluminate. The Furstenberg test (compressing the ipsilateral jugular vein and observing for any change in the lesion) should be negative. Dermoids are usually noncompressible and may be associated with a sinus opening with

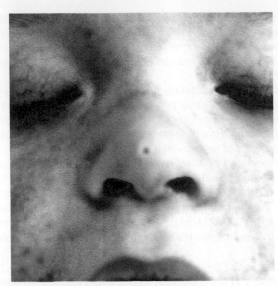

Fig. 8. Pit that is characteristic of a nasal dermoid cyst.

caseous discharge. These lesions do not change in size when straining or compressing vessels and do not transilluminate. They can also have intracranial extensions (**Table 1**).

CT is helpful for bony anatomy of the skull base, and an MRI is helpful to image soft tissue connections at the skull base and within the dura and brain (**Figs. 9** and **10**). Nasal endoscopy can be useful to see the extent of the lesion.

Treatment/Surgical Technique/Procedure

Treatment is surgical for these lesions and is usually done early for lesions with an intracranial extension to minimize the risk of infection/meningitis and cosmetic deformity.[17,23,24] Observation is a reasonable option especially for gliomas and dermoids for up to a few years to decrease perioperative risks if there is no intracranial extension and no clinical contraindication. Observation has to be balanced with the risk of enlargement of the mass and deformity of native structures needing further intervention with waiting. Prophylactic antibiotics are not indicated for identified lesions with

Table 1 Characteristics of anterior congenital nasal masses			
Lesion	Encephalocele	Glioma	Dermoid
Contents	Meninges with or without neural tissue	Glial tissue	Skin appendages
Location	Glabella, nasal dorsum, intranasal, occipital	Glabella, nasal dorsum, nasal tip, intranasal	Nasal dorsum with usually a hair or pit
Intracranial communication	Yes	Possible	Possible
Expansion when straining or vessel compression	Yes	No	No

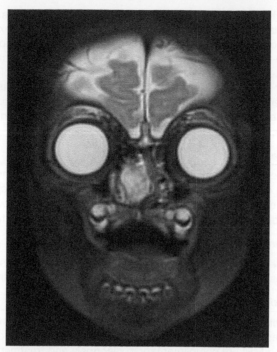

Fig. 9. T2-weighted coronal MRI depicting an intranasal glioma.

intracranial extent before scheduling surgery, because the risk of meningitis is not affected. Preoperatively, however, antibiotics are indicated with an intracranial extent (usually cefazolin and metronidazole or clindamycin). The goal of the surgery is to remove the entire lesion and close off any potential intracranial communication to prevent complications such as a cerebrospinal leak or meningitis. If the lesion is small and intranasal, an endoscopic technique to remove the lesion and its attachments is possible and is the most reasonable approach.[25] Larger lesions that have an intracranial component require a combined approach, with a neurosurgeon performing a craniotomy to resect any intracranial component of the lesion, herniated dura, and neural tissue and close the cerebrospinal fluid leak and an otolaryngologist removing the nasal component of the mass. For the nasal component, possible approaches

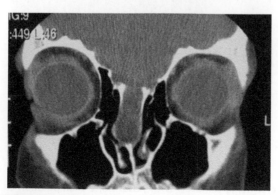

Fig. 10. Coronal CT showing a dermoid cyst with intracranial extension.

include external rhinoplasty, lateral rhinotomy, bicoronal, and midline nasal approach (**Fig. 11**). Rhinoplasty is ideal for nasal septum and nasal dorsum exposure, but the approach does not provide a good access to the glabella. Nasal osteotomies or disarticulation may be needed to follow a stalk that goes to the foramen cecum.[24] The senior author has described a combined closed rhinoplasty/endoscopic approach that can be used for small dermoid lesions that are limited to the nasal dorsum and septum.[26] If a dermoid is extending to the skull base, an option would be to obtain a frozen section of the tract to see if there is extension of the lesion intracranially. If positive, an intracranial approach is used.[19]

Complications/Management

The most common postoperative complications include epistaxis and scar, but the most concerning complications are CSF leak, meningitis, or hydrocephalus. Reoperation may be necessary with persistent problems that do not resolve with conservative measures or medical management. There is a recurrent rate of 4% to 10%.[17]

Postoperative Care

Wound care is necessary for any external scars to prevent infection. Pain control is helpful for successful healing and avoidance of straining and potential complication.

Summary/Discussion

A congenital midline nasal mass should never be biopsied before diagnostic imaging is performed to assess anatomy and study the intracranial extent/communication of the lesion. CT and MRI are complimentary in diagnosis and treatment, and both modalities may be necessary. Clinical examination features can distinguish one lesion from another. Generally, early surgical treatment allows for avoidance of infection and improved cosmesis although urgent surgery is rarely necessary.

NASOLACRIMAL DUCT CYSTS

Nasolacrimal duct cysts or dacryocystoceles can also present as an intranasal mass that causes nasal obstruction. There is aberrant development of the nasolacrimal system, usually at the distal valve into the nasal cavity. Infants with airway distress from bilateral nasolacrimal cysts may need urgent surgery. Thirty percent of all neonates

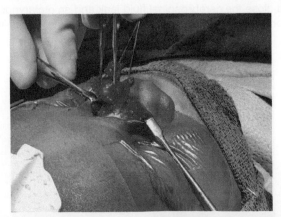

Fig. 11. Dermoid cyst being removed with nasal bone manipulation to follow the stalk. (*Courtesy of* Kara K. Prickett, MD, Emory University School of Medicine, Atlanta, GA.)

have some nasolacrimal duct obstruction at birth.[17] Symptomatic cysts occur rarely, because most of these resolve without treatment.

Anatomy

Canalization of the lacrimal duct begins adjacent to the lacrimal sac and progresses inferiorly. The valve of Hasner is the distal opening of the duct into the nasal cavity and the site that is usually obstructed in these cases. Persistent occlusion at the distal opening or failed maturation of the tract can result in formation of a cyst. Nasal obstruction with respiratory distress is seen when large bilateral cysts fill the inferior meatus of the infant nose.[27]

Diagnosis

Anterior rhinoscopy or nasal endoscopy can show a cystic mass in the inferior meatus. There can be some swelling by the medial canthus of the eye, with or without epiphora. When bilateral and large, respiratory distress is seen. The inferior turbinate may be displaced medially and superiorly by these cysts. CT scans will show a dilated nasolacrimal duct, displaced inferior turbinate, and/or an intranasal cyst (**Fig. 12**). Ophthalmology evaluation is indicated to evaluate the lacrimal system and potentially assist in surgery.

Treatment/Surgical Technique/Procedure

Conservative management can be used with warm compresses and lacrimal massage to try to improve nasolacrimal drainage.[28] When there is respiratory compromise or

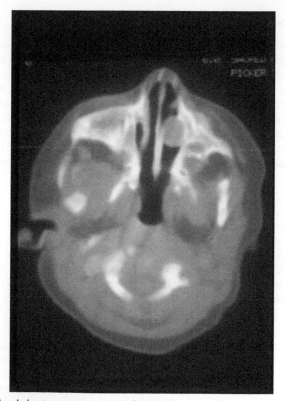

Fig. 12. Nasolacrimal duct cyst seen on axial CT scan.

infection, surgical intervention is preferred.[27] The cyst is marsupialized through a transnasal endoscopic approach either with a microdebrider or with otologic/rhinologic instruments. An ophthalmologist will often probe the lacrimal system and may on occasion leave a lacrimal stent to maintain patency of the lacrimal system. The stents, if placed, are usually removed within a few weeks.

Complications/Management

Complications are rarely seen. Epistaxis is the most common immediate risk that can be controlled with topical decongestants and pressure. Packing is needed rarely. The cysts can recur if the marsupialization was not adequate. Infection and function of the lacrimal system can be affected with surgery as well.

Postoperative Care

Usually intranasal saline is recommended to prevent crusting.

Summary/Discussion

Diagnosis of nasolacrimal duct cysts should be based on examination findings and history. Epiphora, eye crusting, and nasal obstruction suggests the diagnosis. CT scan and nasal endoscopy will confirm the diagnosis. Ophthalmology evaluation and assistance is helpful to ensure functioning of the lacrimal system, especially intraoperatively and postoperatively. Earlier symptoms dictate earlier response.

CONGENITAL NASAL SEPTAL DEVIATION

Neonatal nasal septal deviation is another condition that may lead to respiratory distress. Although nasal septal deviations may be associated with syndromes or a cleft lip/palate deformity, the authors focus on nasal septal deformities found in the absence of these conditions. The incidence of neonatal nasal and septal deviation has been reported between 0.6% and 31%.[29] It is thought to be a result of intrauterine nasal compression or trauma during delivery. Dislocation of the septal cartilage from the maxillary groove is the most commonly noted deviation at birth. Beyond the neonatal period, nasal and septal deviation may lead to compromised nasal breathing, impaired cosmesis, sinusitis, epistaxis, eustachian tube dysfunction, and other health issues.

Anatomy

The anterior portion of the nasal septum is composed of cartilage that is projecting from the face in utero. Because of this projection and the forces in utero, the nose is subject to some trauma and can result in deviation. A dislocation of the cartilage from the maxillary groove may result in an external nasal deformity or at the level of the ethmoid or vomer bones. Internal deformities are due to forces on the skull in utero and may not be as noticeable.[29,30]

Diagnosis

Nasal septal deviations can be suspected in cases of nasal discharge, noisy breathing, respiratory compromise, poor feeding, and traumatic delivery. Most deviations are evident on simple inspection of nasal symmetry supplemented by anterior rhinoscopy. Nasal endoscopy can be used to confirm and see if there are any posterior deviations and rule out other abnormalities mentioned in this article.

Treatment/Surgical Technique/Procedure

Observation of the nasal septal deformities is certainly an option, because the deformity and symptoms may resolve in mild cases without intervention. Sorri and colleagues[31] did not find any significant differences over 8 years in those that were corrected early, noncorrected, and control subjects. When a significant, symptomatic septal deviation is noted within the first few days of life, closed reduction can be done at bedside with a variety of techniques, including the use of a curved hemostat shielded with rubber catheters, if possible. An 11-year follow-up of 49 children showed satisfactory anatomic and functional findings in 46 children.[32]

Complications/Management

Recurrence or persistence of the nasal deformity is always a concern even with early reduction. Epistaxis is likely the most common complication related to septal procedures and can be controlled with pressure/decongestants.

Postoperative Care

None.

Summary

Neonatal septal deviations are usually related to intrauterine or delivery-related trauma. Early identification can be done with rhinoscopy or endoscopy. If symptomatic, closed reduction is certainly a reasonable and successful option in most cases. Observation can certainly be used if not symptomatic.

Best Practices

What is the current practice?

- History and physical examination to determine cause of nasal obstruction
- Noncontrast CT scan for planning/confirmation in choanal atresia and pyriform aperture stenosis
- CT and MRI are helpful in determining nature and course of intranasal masses and determining any intracranial connection
- Avoid biopsy of nasal masses before imaging is done
- Intracranial connection with nasal masses and respiratory/feeding compromise require earlier surgical intervention

What changes in current practice is likely to improve outcomes?

- Recognition of diseases and syndromes associated with the discussed nasal anomalies
- Appropriate analysis of imaging to determine the appropriate approach to a lesion and any consultations needed
- Careful dissection of skull base tracts for any masses to rule out intracranial connection

Clinical algorithm

Major recommendations

- History and physical examination to determine cause of nasal obstruction
- Imaging necessary before intervention on any nasal masses
- Earlier intervention in masses with intracranial extension to avoid meningitis/deformity
- Observation can be done in other cases

- Workup for associated abnormalities is usually warranted with nasal anomalies to achieve the appropriate clinical outcome
- Consultation with ophthalmology for nasolacrimal duct cysts
- Consultation with neurosurgery for intracranial extent of nasal masses/lesions

Summary

Because of neonates being obligate nasal breathers, congenital nasal deformities and masses can result in respiratory distress and urgent otolaryngology consultation. History and physical examination in children with nasal deformities/masses will help direct further workup and management. Earlier treatment is usually dictated by respiratory/feeding status or intracranial connection to any nasal lesions. Other lesions may be observed. The main goals of any procedure to address these lesions are to allow adequate nasal airflow, avoid complications associated with the lesions, and remove any masses/lesions safely without recurrence. Close follow-up is needed to ensure the best clinical outcomes.

REFERENCES

1. Miller MJ, Martin RJ, Carlo WA, et al. Oral breathing in newborn infants. J Pediatr 1985;107(3):465–9.
2. Kwong KM. Current updates on choanal atresia. Front Pediatr 2015;3(52):1–7.
3. Corrales CE, Koltai PJ. Choanal atresia: current concepts and controversies. Curr Opin Otolaryngol Head Neck Surg 2009;17:466–70.
4. Cedin AC, Atallah AN, Andriolo RB, et al. Surgery for congenital choanal atresia (review). Cochrane Database Syst Rev 2012;(2):CD008993.
5. Brihaye P, Delpierre I, DeVille A, et al. Comprehensive management of congenital choanal atresia. Int J Pediatr Otorhinolaryngol 2017;98:9–18.
6. Bedwell JR, Choi SS. Are stents necessary after choanal atresia repair? Laryngoscope 2012;122:2365–6.
7. Stapleton AL, Manning S. Choanal atresia/pyriform aperture stenosis. In: Myers EN, Snyderman CH, editors. Operative otolaryngology: head and neck surgery, vol. 189, 3rd edition. Philadelphia: Elsevier; 2018. p. 1329–31.
8. Tate JR, Sykes J. Congenital nasal pyriform aperture stenosis. Otolaryngol Clin North Am 2009;42:521–5.
9. Adil E, Huntley C, Choudhary A, et al. Congenital nasal obstruction; clinical and radiologic review. Eur J Pediatr 2012;171:641–50.
10. Merea VS, Lee AHY, Peron DL, et al. CPAS; surgical approach with combined sublabial bone resection and inferior turbinate reduction without stents. Laryngoscope 2015;125:1460–4.
11. Collares MVM, Tovo ASH, Duarte DW, et al. Novel treatment of neonates with congenital nasal pyriform aperture stenosis. Laryngoscope 2015;125:2816–9.
12. Wine TM, Dedhia K, Chi DH. Congenital nasal pyriform aperture stenosis; is there a role for nasal dilation. JAMA Otolaryngol Head Neck Surg 2014;140(4):352–6.
13. Gonik NJ, Cheng J, Lesser M, et al. Patient selection in congenital pyriform aperture stenosis repair-14 year experience and systematic review of literature. Int J Pediatr Otorhinolaryngol 2015;79:235–9.
14. Wormold R, Hinton-Bayre A, Bumbak P, et al. Congenital nasal pyriform aperture stenosis 5.7mm or less is associated with surgical intervention; a pooled case series. Int J Pediatr Otorhinolaryngol 2015;79:1802–5.

15. Laurence KM, James N, Miller MH, et al. Double-blind randomized controlled trial of folate treatment before conception to prevent recurrence of neural-tube defects. Br Med J (Clin Res Ed) 1981;282:1509–11.
16. Tirumandas M, Sharma A, Gbenimacho I, et al. Nasal encephaloceles: a review of etiology, pathophysiology, clinical presentations, diagnosis, treatment, and complications. Childs Nerv Syst 2013;29(5):739–44.
17. Elluru RG. Congenital malformations of the nose and nasopharynx. In: Lesperance MM, Flint PW, editors. Cummings pediatric otolaryngology. Philadelphia: Elsevier Saunders; 2014. p. 134–45.
18. Mucaj S, Ugurel MS, Dedushi K, et al. Role of MRI in diagnosis of ruptured intracranial dermoid cyst. Acta Inform Med 2017;25(2):141–4.
19. Herrington H, Adil E, Moritz E, et al. Update on current evaluation and management of pediatric nasal dermoid. Laryngoscope 2016;126:2151–60.
20. Hoving EW. Nasal encephaloceles. Childs Nerv Syst 2000;16:702.
21. Rahbar R, Resto VA, Robson CD, et al. Nasal glioma and encephalocele: diagnosis and management. Laryngoscope 2003;113:2069–77.
22. Bradley PJ, Singh SD. Nasal glioma. J Laryngol Otol 1965;99:247.
23. Sandler AL, Goodrich JT. Encephaloceles, meningoceles, and cranial dermal sinus tracts. In: Winn HR, editor. Youmans and winn neurological surgery, vol. 187, 7th edition. Philadelphia: Elsevier; 2017. p. 1505–17.
24. Wine TM. Midline nasal masses. In: Myers EN, Snyderman CH, editors. Operative otolaryngology: head and neck surgery, vol. 190, 3rd edition. Philadelphia: Elsevier; 2018. p. 1332–40.
25. Kanowitz SH, Bernstein JM. Pediatric meningoencephaloceles and nasal obstruction: a case for endoscopic repair. Int J Pediatr Otorhinolaryngol 2006; 70(12):2087–92.
26. Turner JH, Tunkel DE, Boahene DK. Endoscopic-assisted, closed rhinoplasty approach for excision of nasoglabellar dermoid cysts. Laryngoscope 2010; 120(11):2223–6.
27. Wong R, VanderVeen D. Presentation and management of congenital dacryocystocele. Pediatrics 2008;122:e1108–12.
28. Cunningham MJ. Endoscopic management of pediatric nasolacrimal anomalies. Otolaryngol Clin North Am 2006;39(5):1059–74, viii–ix.
29. Harugop AS, Mudhol RS, Hajare PS, et al. Prevalence of nasal septal deviation in new-borns and its precipitating factors: a cross-sectional study. Indian J Otolaryngol Head Neck Surg 2012;64(3):248–51.
30. Emami AJ, Brodsky L, Pizzuto M. Neonatal septoplasty: case report and review of the literature. Int J Pediatr Otorhinolaryngol 1996;35(3):271–5.
31. Sorri M, Laitakari K, Vainio-Mattila J, et al. Immediate correction of congenital nasal deformities; follow up of 8 years. Int J Pediatr Otorhinolaryngol 1990; 19(3):277–83.
32. Tasca I, Compadretti GC. Immediate correction of nasal septal dislocation in newborns: long-term results. Am J Rhinol 2004;18(1):47–51.

Congenital Neck Masses

Lourdes Quintanilla-Dieck, MD[a],*, Edward B. Penn Jr, MD[b]

KEYWORDS

- Pediatric • Congenital • Neck mass • Neck lesion

KEY POINTS

- There is a broad differential for congenital neck masses, because they can be either developmental or neoplastic. They can also be cystic, solid, or of vascular origin.
- Presentation and physical examination can help narrow the differential diagnosis and guide prompt referral to the appropriate pediatric specialists.
- Imaging plays an essential role in diagnosis; ultrasonography, MRI, and computed tomography can all be used and each has advantages and disadvantages.

INTRODUCTION

Congenital head and neck masses are by definition present at birth, although they may not be diagnosed until a later stage of life.[1] Perinatologists and pediatricians may encounter a child with a neck mass and, given the wide variety of possible causes, it is important to use the history and presentation to subsequently narrow the differential diagnosis and make an appropriate referral to a pediatric specialist. Congenital masses can be a developmental anomaly of cystic, solid, or vascular nature. Rarely, they are neoplastic, although only 5% of pediatric neoplasms occur in the head and neck.[2]

The history related to the lesion as well as a thorough physical examination of the head and neck are essential for diagnosis. The history should include onset, duration, changes in appearance or symptoms, presence of multiple lesions, associated pain or dysphagia, and leakage of fluid. The presence of other syndromic features should be investigated. A detailed physical examination can be helpful in narrowing the possibilities. Midline neck masses may constitute thyroglossal duct cysts, dermoid or epidermoid cysts, cervical clefts, or teratomas. Lateral neck masses are more likely to be branchial cleft anomalies, lymphatic or vascular malformations, or thyroid nodules.[2]

Disclosure: The authors have no disclosures or conflicts of interest to disclose.
[a] Department of Otolaryngology Head and Neck Surgery, Oregon Health & Science University, 3181 Southwest Sam Jackson Park Road, PV-01, Portland, OR 97239, USA; [b] Department of General Surgery, Greenville Health System, Greenville ENT Associates, 200 Patewood Drive Suite B400, Greenville, SC 29615, USA
* Corresponding author.
E-mail address: quintani@ohsu.edu

In addition, imaging plays an essential role in defining the nature and extent of the mass. A systematic approach to imaging masses includes determining the primary site of origin, which anatomic spaces of the head or neck are involved, and the characteristic imaging features.[1] Ultrasonography (US) and MRI are the imaging modalities of choice in the pediatric population for congenital lesions.[1,3] Computed tomography (CT) scanning is another valuable modality that can also be indicated, but its inherent ionizing radiation exposure leads to a more restricted use in children. These 3 imaging modalities each have advantages and disadvantages (Table 1).

PRENATAL DIAGNOSIS OF HEAD AND NECK MASSES

Modern imaging modalities enable prenatal diagnosis of many neck masses. Large fetal neck masses may cause significant effects because of compression on surrounding cervical and facial structures.[4] For example, compression on the tracheoesophageal complex can lead to impaired fetal swallowing, polyhydramnios, airway obstruction, and preterm labor. Ultimately, depending on the severity, this can lead to neonatal hypoxia and death. Deformity of developing cervicofacial structures can also occur. Fetal head and neck masses can initially be diagnosed with ultrasonography, but fetal MRI can be very helpful in delineating specific anatomic findings and permitting adequate prenatal counseling and planning.

Congenital head and neck masses require detailed planning of perinatal management, especially if there is any sign of airway obstruction, which is usually the most life-threatening factor at birth. For fetuses at risk of airway compromise at birth, an ex utero intrapartum treatment (EXIT) procedure provides a safe delivery option to stabilize the infant during transition from fetal to neonatal physiology. This strategy has gained wide acceptance at a large number of centers for the management of fetal and impending neonatal cardiorespiratory compromise.[5] Its main purpose is to give time at delivery for airway management and resuscitation of the infant while remaining on placental oxygen support. However, preprocedural consent is important; previous studies show that women undergoing an EXIT procedure have higher blood loss and increased risk of postoperative wound complications compared with those having a cesarean delivery.[6] In one recent retrospective series, 4 out of 35 infants with prenatally diagnosed neck masses died shortly after birth. Two had massive cervical teratomas and died of airway obstruction when an EXIT procedure could not be done, one because of precipitous preterm birth and another because of placental abruption.[4] EXIT was performed successfully in 18 of 31 (58%) infants with giant neck masses; most were lymphatic malformations and teratomas. The EXIT procedure can be considered in any prenatally diagnosed situation in which possible need for neonatal cardiopulmonary resuscitation is anticipated. As such, prompt referral to a tertiary center with all required specialties is important in this scenario.

CONGENITAL CYSTIC MASSES
Thyroglossal Duct Cysts

The thyroid gland starts to form in the third week in utero from endoderm of the first and second pharyngeal pouches.[7] Starting on the pharyngeal floor, it descends to and around the developing hyoid bone and eventually occupies its final position in the lower anterior neck overlying the larynx.[2,3,7] As the thyroid anlage migrates caudally, a tract forms the thyroglossal duct. During the fifth to eighth week of gestation, the duct obliterates and proximally leaves the foramen cecum as its remnant at

Table 1
Characteristics of the most common imaging modalities for neck masses

Characteristic	US	MRI	CT
Advantages	High-resolution image quality Noninvasive Inexpensive Readily available Does not require sedation Real-time character allows evaluation of mobility and compressibility of the mass	High-quality evaluation of soft tissues and deep lesions with excellent soft tissue contrast	Fast and readily available, which can be useful in the emergency setting
Disadvantages	Limited in evaluating tissues deep to bony structures	High cost Infants and young children may require general anesthesia Longer acquisition times; however, currently available fast-sequence MRI techniques can be done in some cases	Long-term risks of ionizing radiation, especially in children
Details of soft tissues	Can differentiate well between solid and cystic masses Identifies calcifications Doppler US can identify vascular flow and analysis of the spectral blood flow waveforms can help differentiate between types of vascular anomalies	Detailed soft tissue evaluation, more specific than US, especially with deep lesions Optimal visualization of displaced anatomic spaces, vascular anatomy, and neural elements Resolution enhanced by gadolinium-based contrast agent administration Delayed contrast-enhanced sequences can characterize vascular masses and malformations	Preferred for acute diagnostic work-up of infections or abscesses in the neck
Details of bony structures	Poor	Poor	Best for evaluating bony structures
Radiation exposure?	No	No	Yes

Data from Dremmen MHG, Tekes A, Mueller S, et al. Lumps and bumps of the neck in children-neuroimaging of congenital and acquired lesions. J Neuroimaging 2016;26:562–80; and Travinh E, Yeom KW, lv M. Imaging neck masses in the neonate and young infant. Semin Ultrasound CT MR 2015;36:120–37.

the base of tongue.[7] The distal remnant forms the pyramidal lobe of the thyroid gland. A thyroglossal duct cyst (TGDC) forms when this tract persists and fails to obliterate. This embryologic migration of the thyroid gland is essential to understand the possible locations where TGDCs can arise: anywhere between the base of tongue and the thyroid gland; the most common location is adjacent to the hyoid bone (66%).[7]

TGDCs are the most common congenital pediatric neck mass, followed by branchial cleft anomalies and dermoid cysts.[7] Two-thirds of patients with TGDCs are diagnosed before 30 years of age, and more than 50% of these are clinically apparent before 10 years of age. They may present as asymptomatic neck masses or, if they get secondarily infected, they may appear for the first time as a swollen and painful mass. At times these masses rupture spontaneously and develop a draining sinus, which may occur after an upper respiratory infection. On examination, TGDCs are most easily seen with neck extension and elevate with swallowing and tongue protrusion given their relationship to the hyoid bone.

The best modality for imaging TGDCs in children is ultrasonography, which can delineate the position of the cyst, its relationship to the hyoid bone, and the presence of normal thyroid gland tissue. The presence of normal thyroid gland tissue is important before undergoing surgical excision, to ensure that the surgeon does not remove the entirety of the patient's thyroid tissue. It also helps rule out a lingual thyroid. The ultrasonography features of an uncomplicated TGDC are thin walls, anechoic, heterogeneous with internal septae, and presence of solid components (**Fig. 1**). If they have been infected they can have a thick wall, or they can be hypoechoic in the presence of hemorrhage.[8] Fewer than 1% of TGDCs develop malignancy, which is more common in adults but has been reported in children as young as 6 years of age.[7]

The Sistrunk procedure, first described in 1920, is the recommended surgical treatment of TGDCs in order to ensure complete removal. This surgery involves removal of the cyst and any associated tract as well as the middle portion of the hyoid bone (**Fig. 2**). Failure to remove the hyoid bone results in high recurrence rates.[2,7] Patients with infected, draining sinuses are also at increased risk for recurrence.

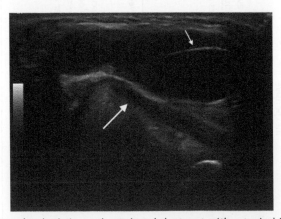

Fig. 1. Ultrasonography depicting a thyroglossal duct cyst with a typical internal septation (*small arrow*) overlying the laryngeal framework, specifically the thyroid cartilage (*large arrow*).

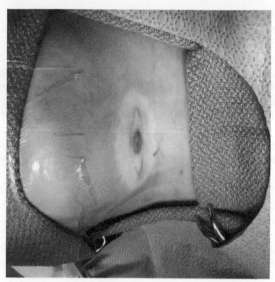

Fig. 2. Planned incision for a thyroglossal duct cyst removal via Sistrunk procedure. Note location in upper midline neck, adjacent to hyoid bone, and draining sinus tract to the skin in the middle of planned incision.

Branchial Cleft Anomalies

The tissues of the neck are derived from branchial arches, which are separated externally by grooves and internally by pharyngeal pouches. The branchial arches are covered with ectoderm on the surface, whereas the inside pouches consist of foregut endoderm; mesoderm-derived tissue lies between the two layers.[7] A branchial cleft anomaly results from incomplete or aberrant fusion of 2 adjacent arches.[2] These anomalies can include cysts (isolated epithelial-lined structures lacking connection to the skin or pharynx), sinuses (connecting either the skin or pharynx to a blind pouch in the neck), and fistulas (an open tract between the skin and the pharynx) and have characteristic locations based on the arch they are derived from and their relationship to nerves, arteries, and muscles.[9]

Cysts arising from the first branchial arch constitute about 8% of cervical sinus tracts and cysts.[10] Type I first arch cysts typically open in the preauricular or post-auricular region. The sinus tract usually courses parallel to the external auditory canal, and it can attach to the skin of the external auditory canal or to the tympanic membrane.[2,7] Type I lesions are found lateral to the facial nerve. Type II first arch cysts, by contrast, are medial to the facial nerve.[7] They are located in the anterior neck, superior to the hyoid. The typical course of the type II first arch sinus follows is anterior to the hyoid, often through the parotid gland and around the facial nerve.[2] These first arch anomalies may be asymptomatic, but some patients present with discomfort of the cervical, parotid, or auricular regions. A pitlike depression close to the angle of the mandible may be identified and can lead to drainage if infected.

Cysts of the second branchial arch are the most common, and account for 90% to 95% of cervical cysts.[2,7] If derived from the second branchial pouch, these anomalies can form fistulous tracts and connect the palatine tonsil to the lateral neck skin at the anterior border of the sternocleidomastoid muscle. Examination reveals a skin pit in this location. Alternatively, if derived from the second branchial cleft, they can enter the supratonsillar fossa and pass adjacent to the glossopharyngeal and hypoglossal nerves. If these pits are found bilaterally, the child should be screened for branchio-oto-renal syndrome because there may also be underlying hearing loss and kidney disease. These cysts can be located in proximity to the carotid sheath, at times passing between the internal and external carotid arteries.[7] If a skin pit is present, it is located along the anterior border of the sternocleidomastoid muscle. Patients may present with acute enlargement of these cysts or superinfection, frequently during an upper respiratory tract infection. Depending on the location and size, this enlargement can lead to respiratory compromise, torticollis, or dysphagia.[7]

Cysts of the third and fourth branchial arches are very uncommon, comprising less than 2% of branchial arch anomalies.[2] These cysts typically have sinus tracts that course deep into the anterior cervical structures and thyroid gland and terminate in the pyriform fossa. If these anomalies get secondarily infected, they may present as suppurative thyroiditis in children. If they enlarge rapidly with infection, they can also present with tracheal compression or airway compression in young children.[7]

For all of these cysts, surgical excision is the mainstay of treatment. Preoperative imagine is often used to plan the surgical approach and anticipate potential complications. Cysts and sinuses that are not resected have a high risk of infection. In addition, incomplete resection may result in higher rates of recurrence.[7] Their anatomic location may imply certain precautions during surgery. For example, for type II first branchial arch cysts, a superficial parotidectomy may be required for full excision of the cyst and sinus and to avoid damage to the facial nerve. For the third and fourth branchial arch cysts, endoscopic examination of the pyriform fossa is important in order to identify the internal sinus opening, most commonly on the left side.[2] Fourth arch anomalies require ipsilateral hemithyroidectomy for complete excision of the tract.[7]

Dermoid and Epidermoid Cysts

Dermoid cysts are rare, and studies have shown an incidence of 3 per 10,000 general pediatric patients.[11] Epidermoid cysts are derived solely from ectoderm, whereas dermoid cysts are benign neoplasms derived from ectoderm and mesoderm. Epidermoid cysts are normally found superficially in subcutaneous tissues. Dermoid cysts form from epithelial remnants found along embryonic fusion lines. They are composed of keratinizing squamous epithelium as well as occasional dermal derivatives such as hair follicles, fibroadipose tissue, smooth muscle, and sweat and sebaceous glands.[11]

Only 40% of congenital dermoid cysts are noted in the newborn period, and about 70% are diagnosed by 5 years of age.[11] These cysts grow slowly during the first few years of life, and then remain largely unchanged in later years. Approximately 7% present in the head and neck, and the most common site is the outer third of the eyebrow.[3,11] On the neck, the 2 most frequent locations are in the parahyoid region (thereby mimicking TGDCs) and, in the suprasternal area, between the strap muscles and traveling down onto the trachea. When dermoids are in the midline of the nasal area, they may be associated with dysraphism or have intracranial extension. The most common of midline dermoid cysts are nasal dermoids, which develop during ossification of the frontonasal plate and result from failure of closure of the neuropore (**Fig. 3**). This location accounts for 12.6% of dermal cysts in the head and neck.[3] Nasal

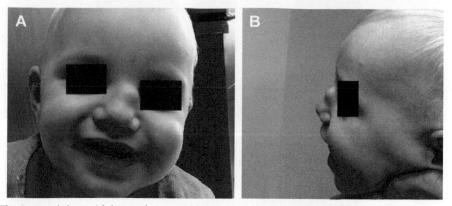

Fig. 3. Nasal dermoid, located on nasal bridge just left of midline. (*A*) Frontal view. (*B*) Profile view.

dermoids present as swelling over the nasal dorsum, anywhere from the glabella to the nasal tip (**Fig. 4**). Often they are associated with a sinus opening or punctum, and they may present with recurrent infections.

The management of dermoid cysts depends on their location. Most dermoids require only simple excision, although at times the midline dermoids can travel through deeper tissues and may require a more extensive surgery (**Fig. 5**). Midline nasal dermoids have a risk of intracranial extension and require imaging to rule this out. The nasal dermoid requires dissection down to the upper lateral nasal cartilages and/or nasal bones and may require a combined approach with neurosurgery if intracranial extension is suspected. For all dermoid cysts, every effort should be made to remove the entire cyst without rupture of the cyst wall and spillage of contents,[2] because this

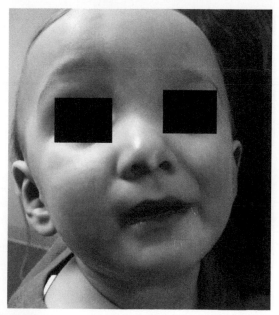

Fig. 4. Nasal tip dermoid.

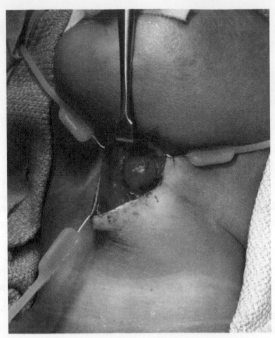

Fig. 5. Intraoperative view during removal of a dermoid cyst located in the upper midline neck, mimicking a thyroglossal duct cyst in its location.

can lead to recurrence (**Fig. 6**). Dermoids may be attached to underlying periosteum and require removal of the involved segment of periosteal attachment. Another option is observation, because infections are uncommon; however, these lesions will continue to grow and are likely to ultimately require excision.

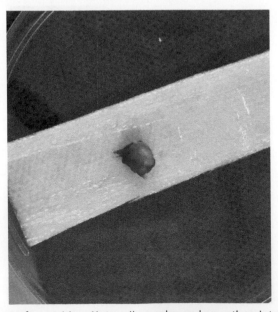

Fig. 6. Dermoid cyst after excision. Note yellow color and smooth uninterrupted wall.

Thymic Cysts

The thymus forms from the third branchial pouch and descends to the mediastinum through the thymopharyngeal duct, traveling lateral to the thyroid gland.[12] It is along this pathway that a thymic cyst can arise: from the angle of the mandible, adjacent to the carotid sheath, to the thoracic inlet. About two-thirds of patients present in the first decade of life, and most of these lesions are asymptomatic.[12] Alternatively, they can present as gradually enlarging, soft and compressible cervical masses that may extend into the mediastinum. When very large, they can present with compressive symptoms. Complete surgical resection is the treatment of choice.

Bronchogenic Cysts

Cervical bronchogenic cysts are extremely rare. Anomalous foregut development is suspected to play a role in their cause. They have been reported in infants as well as in adults. Their usual location is in the suprasternal notch, presternum, shoulder, neck, base of tongue, infraclavicular area, or chin. They can extend into the mediastinum. These cysts may present as masses that fluctuate in size but usually enlarge proportionally to body growth. Symptoms can include dyspnea, cyanosis, or dysphagia caused by local traction or compression on surrounding structures. They can also get infected and therefore present as neck abscesses.[12]

Foregut Duplication Cysts

Foregut duplication cysts (FDCs) of the oral cavity are very rare. Before 2004, only 21 reported cases of these existed.[11] The embryologic foregut gives rise to the pharynx, lower respiratory tract, esophagus, stomach, duodenum, and hepatobiliary tract. Duplication cysts occur anywhere along the alimentary tract from the oral cavity to the rectum. Midgut duplications are most common, and foregut duplications account for one-third. Oral cavity duplication cysts constitute 0.3% of all duplication cysts.[11] FDCs are typically diagnosed in asymptomatic neonates and small children and may result in swallowing difficulties or, most concerning, in airway obstruction. The first step in management is securing the airway. At times, intubation or a tracheostomy are required. There have been reported cases of FDCs identified in utero that have required an EXIT procedure to secure the airway.[13] The mainstay of treatment is surgical excision.

CONGENITAL SOLID MASSES
Ectopic Thyroid

Although rare, this can present as stridor and airway embarrassment at birth and in the perinatal period. This lesion may be misdiagnosed as a TGDC so imaging is prudent to determine whether the thyroid gland is present in its normal location. This condition affects girls more than boys (female/male, 4:1). Incidence varies between 1:3000 and 1:10,000 and although usually asymptomatic, in approximately 75% of cases, ectopic thyroid tissue represents the only functional thyroid tissue. This condition is a result of the lack of caudal migration of the thyroid gland. Although most commonly present in the tongue, other locations include the sublingual space, suprahyoid region, mediastinum, precardial sac, heart, breast, upper esophagus, and even in the abdomen.[14] Differential should also include lymphatic malformations, thyroglossal duct cysts, angiomas, adenomas, fibromas, and lipomas.[14]

Evaluation of ectopic thyroid should include imaging via US, and CT and/or MRI. To determine whether this remains the only functioning thyroid tissue, a thyroid scan with technetium 99m sodium should be used. Factors that should be discussed before treatment should include age of the patient; location and size of the lesion; effect of lesion on surrounding structures; state of the thyroid gland; and the presence of complications such as ulceration, hemorrhage, cystic degeneration, or concern for malignancy.[15–17]

Patients that are asymptomatic require no treatment as long as they are euthyroid, although patients should be followed to avoid development of complications such as malignant transformation. Thyroid replacement hormone therapy may produce a slow reduction in size of the mass. Ablative radioactive therapy is an option for nonsurgical candidates, although attempts to avoid this treatment in children and young adults are paramount because of damaging effects to gonads or other organs.[17–19] Surgical treatment, transoral or external, should also be considered based on complicating factors discussed earlier in addition to local symptoms.

Teratomas

Teratomas are germ cell neoplasms that can occur in the cervical and craniofacial regions. They consist of all 3 embryonic layers (ectoderm, mesoderm, and endoderm). Teratomas affecting the head and neck account for 2% to 5% of all germ cell neoplasms, with cervical teratomas representing the most common location.[20–23] They are classified based on location in which they occur: gonadal or extragonadal. Orbital, nasopharyngeal, oropharyngeal, temporal bone, infratemporal fossa, and intracranial locations have also been reported. Teratomas in utero can lead to pulmonary hypoplasia, feeding issues, along with respiratory distress at birth caused by obstruction of the aerodigestive tract. Obstruction can also lead to abnormal intrauterine deglutination and subsequent polyhydramnios.[21] Resultant respiratory distress may necessitate need for an EXIT procedure. Obstruction is overcome via intubation or tracheostomy with a plan for complete surgical excision at this time or a later date.[22] A special consideration should be made for teratomas affecting the palate, termed an epignathus. This teratoma is the most common craniofacial teratoma in newborns. They are typically attached to the palate via a stalk and, once resected, imaging is paramount to determine persistence of disease at the skull base and parapharyngeal areas.[22]

These solid tumors usually present as well-circumscribed masses.[20] They are variable in consistency, with both cystic and solid areas, and are also made up of cartilage, bone, and pigmented areas. On histology, they are classified into immature and mature teratomas. The mature teratomas commonly affect the pediatric population and consist of mature skin, hair, fat, tissue, cartilage, bone, and glands. Immature teratomas contain immature elements.[20,22,24]

Radiologic imaging may consist of calcified tissue within the mass, which can be suggestive of a teratoma. Prenatal US can aid in identification of involved sites and in the differential diagnosis. When a teratoma is concerned, fetal MRI can also establish proximity to, or involvement of, critical structures.

Although securing the airway and providing respiratory support is the primary initial goal, early surgical excision, when feasible, can aid in prevention of infectious sequelae, coagulopathies, and bleeding. There is a 5% risk of malignancy with increasing age at resection. Surgical resection is often difficult because teratomas frequently infiltrate adjacent tissues. The surgical risk of mortality may be as high as 15%.[22,25]

Tumor recurrence is high if resection is incomplete, although complete resection with clear margins may be challenging because of involvement of critical structures. Tumor recurrence may be monitored by alpha fetoprotein levels, although it is unclear how long these patients should be followed clinically and radiographically.[20,22]

Vascular Anomalies

Vascular anomalies represent a complex and broad range of head and neck masses and can be seen in up to 4.5% of the pediatric population.[26,27] Although many of these tumors are present at birth, some mature and enlarge over the first year of life, whereas others have the potential to immediately hinder perinatal development. These tumors commonly affect the head and neck and many present in the perinatal period can lead to significant morbidity because of involvement and mass effect of adjacent structures.

Infantile hemangiomas

Infantile hemangiomas (IHs) are vascular tumors. They are seen in 4% to 10% of infants and represent the most common vascular anomaly. They are usually present before the age of 1 year, with 60% of these present in the head and neck. IHs are associated with low birth weight and premature infants. In addition, the incidence of hemangiomas in infants less than 1000 g is up to 30%.[26–28] They are also more common in white infants, low birth weight infants, and multiple gestations. Other risk factors include placental abnormalities and women whose mothers underwent amniocentesis or chorionic villus sampling.[29] Ultrasonography of these lesions shows a high-flow vascular tumor with numerous vascular channels.

The natural history of these lesions involves 3 stages: an early proliferative phase, an involuting phase, and an involuted phase. The proliferative phase is characterized by rapid growth of the abnormal blood vessels during the first 6 months of life and can extend to 10 to 12 months of life. These vessels usually are not present at birth but, during rapid growth, they appear bright red and exophytic. This phase can lead to significant disfigurement, ulceration, and bleeding. By the age of 5 months, most IHs grow to 80% of their potential size. Involution starts around 12 months of age. Approximately 30% of IHs are involuted by 3 years, 50% by 5 years, and some involution lasts up to 10 years of age.[26,30]

Glucose transporter protein type 1 (GLUT-1) is a specific marker for IH, with 97% of IHs testing positive for GLUT-1. Lesions with IH-like characteristics not responding to propranolol treatment demand biopsy testing for GLUT-1 positivity. GLUT-1–negative tumors do not follow typical proliferation or involution staging.[26,31]

Special considerations include patients presenting with 5 or more cutaneous IHs. This situation prompts abdominal imaging (MRI or US) to investigate for liver hemangiomas.[32,33] Segmental facial hemangiomas should be evaluated for PHACE (posterior fossa lesions, hemangiomas, arterial lesions, cardiac abnormalities, and eye abnormalities; **Fig. 7**) syndrome. IHs affecting the "beard" distribution of the lower face need to be assessed carefully for airway involvement. Up to 20% of these patients also have a subglottic hemangioma, which can lead to biphasic stridor, dysphagia, and recurrent croup.[26,32]

Historically, these lesions may have been treated with systemic steroids, intralesional steroid injections, and surgical intervention. In 2008, the US Food and Drug Administration (FDA) approved propranolol as an agent to treat IHs. This medication is now the mainstay of treatment and has shown an excellent side effect profile.[34,35] With the use of propranolol, surgical options have decreased as the initial option for treatment. Note that up to 50% of IHs still need a procedure at some point.[26]

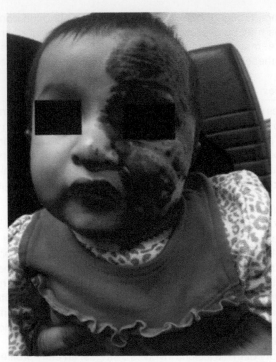

Fig. 7. Patient with PHACE syndrome.

Venous malformations

Venous malformations (VMs) are the third most common vascular anomaly in the head and neck and are present and birth. They typically are compressible masses with over-lying blue or purple skin staining. These lesions expand with dependent drainage such as leaning the patient back and placing the head below the heart and the Valsalva maneuver.[26,36]

On histology, these lesions are made up of numerous aberrant venous channels in communication with each other. Phleboliths are characteristic of VMs, may feel firm to palpation, and may cause severe pain with tenderness. US may better define VMs, which show as well-demarcated lesions containing compressible hypoechoic tubular channels that are low flow. MRI reveals isointensity on T1-weighted sequences and hyperintensity on T2-weighted sequences.[26,36]

Management is usually multimodal and can include any of the following: sclerotherapy, surgery, laser therapy, or a combination of the three. Surgical interven-tion can be straightforward with well-demarcated planes, whereas other VMs may be delicately intertwined with critical structures with irregular borders leading to difficulty in total resection (**Fig. 8**). Mucosal and aerodigestive VMs may be treated with laser therapy, best performed with the neodymium:yttrium-aluminum-garnet laser.[36] Scle-rosing agents, typically alcohol-based agents, may be injected into the lesion under image guidance. Patients may need up to 4 sessions separated by 3 to 12 months in order to fully and therapeutically treat these lesions.[37]

Lymphatic malformations

Lymphatic malformations are low-flow lesions involving the head and neck. Because of the rich supply of lymphatics in this area, these vascular lesions are

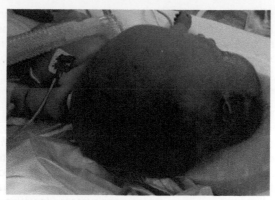

Fig. 8. Patient with large obstructing VM requiring EXIT procedure.

seen in this area 75% of the time. They are classified into microcystic, macrocystic, and mixed. This class of lesion is more likely to lead to perinatal aerodigestive tract obstruction after birth and, as such, may be treated with an EXIT procedure. These lesions are classified into 2 categories: macrocystic lesions have cysts greater than 2 cm in diameter and microcystic lesions have cysts less than 2 cm in diameter.[26,27]

On histology, these lesions, both macrocystic and microcystic, are made up of ectatic, thin-walled, irregularly shaped vessels of heterogenous size.[38,39] Surgically, larger macrocystic disease can be affixed to muscle, bone, and nerve tissue, whereas smaller microcystic disease can be even more involved with these tissues, making complete surgical resection difficult. Microcystic disease is also commonly associated with mucosal disease and both forms can acutely enlarge with viral or bacterial infections affecting the head and neck.

Treatment of lymphatic malformation is often multifactorial and multidisciplinary, which must take into account each individual lesion. As with VMs, sclerotherapy may be used and can consist different sclerosants, such as ethanol, sodium tetradecyl, bleomycin, or doxycycline.[26,37] Laser treatments using CO_2 laser or coblation have also produced excellent results.[26]

Rhabdomyosarcoma

Rhabdomyosarcomas (RMSs) are the most common soft tissue malignancy in the pediatric population, accounting for 50% to 70% of all childhood sarcomas. Up to 43% of patients present at less than 5 years old, which may include the perinatal period. Although most cases are sporadic, there seem to be risk factors, including parental smoking, in utero radiation exposure, advanced maternal age, maternal history of prior spontaneous abortions, and maternal recreational drug use. Several familial syndromes are also associated with an increased risk for RMS: Li-Fraumeni syndrome, Beckwith-Wiedemann syndrome, and Costello syndrome.[40–42]

There are 4 different histopathologic subtypes: embryonal (54%), alveolar (18.5%), undifferentiated (6.5%), and botryoid (4.5%).[43] The most common sites in the head and neck are the nasopharynx, paranasal sinuses, middle ear, and the infratemporal fossa. These sites are considered parameningeal sites. These tumors are aggressive and spread by hematogenous and lymphatic routes. Approximately 13% of patients with lesions involving the head and neck present with distant metastasis.[44]

This lesion is staged by the TNM (tumor, node, metastasis) system and treatment guidelines have been established by the Intergroup Rhabdomyosarcoma Study. Treatment options usually consist of surgical options with additional radiation therapy if resection is incomplete. Nearly all patients receive systemic chemotherapy whether preoperatively or postoperatively.

SUMMARY

When a mass in the head and neck is identified, a broad range of causes should come to mind. The clinical history alone can help distinguish a congenital mass from an acquired one. Furthermore, the exact location of the tumor can narrow the differential diagnoses to 1 or 2. Imaging studies are commonly done for confirmation or to delineate the extent of involvement of adjacent structures, especially in preparation for surgical excision. Some of the most common masses encountered in young children are thyroglossal duct cysts, branchial cleft cysts, and dermoid cysts. Vascular tumors are also common and have a typical presentation. However, the most common masses by far are benign, but it is important to keep in mind malignant causes, which can rarely be congenital. Early diagnosis and referral to subspecialists is key, and their individual treatments can have lifelong consequences.

Best Practices

What is the current practice?

Congenital head/neck mass

- Complete history and physical examination are key for diagnosis.

- Location can point to cause.

- Imaging is usually necessary for confirming cause and determining type and extent of lesion.

- Can be divided into cystic versus solid. Cystic masses most commonly are formed of thyroglossal duct cysts and branchial cleft cysts. Lymphovascular masses are common in the solid category.

  ○ Thyroglossal duct cysts are removed via a Sistrunk procedure, which includes removal of the central portion of the hyoid bone and leads to significantly lower recurrence rates compared with simple excision of the cyst.

  ○ Branchial cleft anomalies comprise cysts, sinuses, and fistulae. Treatment must be tailored to each specific type. Third and fourth branchial cleft cysts can be treated endoscopically, because open excision leads to higher risk of complications in young children.

  ○ One common type of vascular anomaly is hemangioma. Historically, these lesions have been treated with systemic steroids, intralesional steroid injections, and surgical intervention. In 2008, the FDA approved propranolol as a treatment agent, and this medication is now the mainstay of treatment.

What changes in current practice are likely to improve outcomes?

- Prenatal diagnosis of head and neck lesions and the EXIT procedure.

  Current imaging modalities, including ultrasonography and fetal MRI, enable prenatal diagnosis of many neck masses. Large fetal neck masses may cause significant effects because of compression on surrounding cervical and facial structures. For fetuses at risk of airway compromise at birth, an EXIT procedure provides a safe delivery option to stabilize the infant during transition from fetal to neonatal physiology. This strategy has gained wide acceptance for the management of fetal and impending neonatal cardiorespiratory compromise.

Clinical algorithm

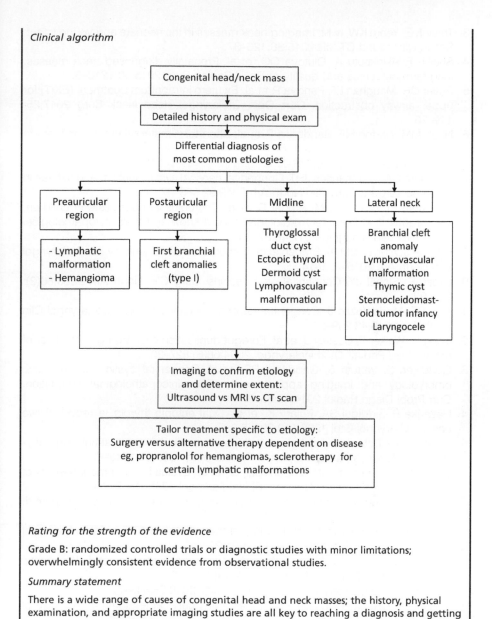

Rating for the strength of the evidence

Grade B: randomized controlled trials or diagnostic studies with minor limitations; overwhelmingly consistent evidence from observational studies.

Summary statement

There is a wide range of causes of congenital head and neck masses; the history, physical examination, and appropriate imaging studies are all key to reaching a diagnosis and getting subspecialty care in a timely fashion.

REFERENCES

1. Dremmen MHG, Tekes A, Mueller S, et al. Lumps and bumps of the neck in children–neuroimaging of congenital and acquired lesions. J Neuroimaging 2016;26:562–80.

2. Goins MR, Beasley MS. Pediatric neck masses. Oral Maxillofacial Surg Clin North Am 2012;24:457–68.

3. Travinh E, Yeom KW, Iv M. Imaging neck masses in the neonate and young infant. Semin Ultrasound CT MR 2015;36:120–37.
4. Sheikh F, Akinkoutu A, Olutoye OO, et al. Prenatally diagnosed neck masses: long-term outcomes and quality of life. J Pediatr Surg 2015;50:1210–3.
5. Butler CR, Maughan EF, Pandya P, et al. Ex utero intrapartum treatment (EXIT) for upper airway obstruction. Curr Opin Otolaryngol Head Neck Surg 2017;25: 119–26.
6. Noah MM, Norton ME, Sandberg P, et al. Short-term maternal outcomes that are associated with the EXIT procedure, as compared with cesarean delivery. Am J Obstet Gynecol 2002;186:773–7.
7. LaRiviere CA, Waldhausen JHT. Congenital cervical cysts, sinuses, and fistulae in pediatric surgery. Surg Clin North Am 2012;92:583–97.
8. Clemente EI, Oyewumi M, Propst E, et al. Thyroglossal duct cysts in children: sonographic features every radiologist should know and their histopathological correlation. Clin Imaging 2017;46:57–64.
9. Prosser JD, Myer CM III. Branchial cleft anomalies and thymic cysts. Otolaryngol Clin North Am 2015;48:1–14.
10. Gross E, Sichel JY. Congenital neck lesions. Surg Clin North Am 2006;86(2): 383–92.
11. Hills SE, Maddalozzo J. Congenital lesions of epithelial origin. Otolaryngol Clin North Am 2015;48:209–23.
12. Kong K, Walker P, Cassey J, et al. Foregut duplication cyst arising in the floor of mouth. Int J Pediatr Otorhinolaryngol 2004;68(6):827–30.
13. Gaddikeri S, Vattoth S, Gaddikeri RS, et al. Congenital cystic neck masses: embryology and imaging appearances, with clinicopathological correlation. Curr Probl Diagn Radiol 2014;43:55–67.
14. Hazarika P, Siddiqui SA, Pujary K, et al. Dual ectopic thyroid: a report of two cases. J Laryngol Otol 1998;112:393–5.
15. Benedetto V. Ectopic thyroid gland in the submandibular region simulating a thyroglossal duct cyst: a case report. J Pediatr Surg 1997;32:1745–6.
16. Williams JD, Scalafani AP, Slupchinskij O, et al. Evaluation and management of the lingual thyroid gland. Ann Otol Rhinol Laryngol 1996;105:312–6.
17. Oomen KP, Modi VK, Maddalozzo J. Thyroglossal duct cyst and ectopic thyroid. Otolaryngol Clin North Am 2015;48:15–27.
18. Danner C, Bodenner D, Breay R. Lingual thyroid: iodine 131: a viable treatment modality revisited. Am J Otolaryngol 2001;22:276–81.
19. Weider DJ, Parker W. Lingual thyroid: review, case reports, and therapeutic guidelines. Ann Otol Rhinol Laryngol 1977;86:841–8.
20. Lakhoo K. Neonatal teratomas. Early Hum Dev 2010;86:643–7.
21. Rosenfield CR, Coln CD, Duenholter JH. Fetal cervical teratoma as a cause of polyhydramnios. Pediatrics 1979;64:176–9.
22. Paradis J, Koltai PJ. Pediatric teratoma and dermoid cysts. Otolaryngol Clin North Am 2015;48:121–36.
23. Coppit GL, Perkins JA, Manning S. Nasopharyngeal teratomas and dermoids: a review of literature and case series. Int J Pediatr Otorhinolaryngol 2000;52: 219–27.
24. Wakhlu AK. Head and neck teratomas in children. Pediatr Surg Int 2000;16: 333–7.
25. Shine NP, Sader C, Gollow I, et al. Congenital cervical teratomas: diagnostic, management, and postoperative variability. Arch Otolaryngol Head Neck Surg 1994;120(4):444–9.

26. Hoff SR, Rastatter JC, Richter GT. Head and neck vascular lesions. Otolaryngol Clin North Am 2015;48:29–45.
27. Buckmiller L, Richter G, Suen J. Diagnosis and management of hemangiomas and vascular malformations of the head and neck. Oral Dis 2010;16(5):405–18.
28. Mulliken J, Glowacki J. Hemangiomas and vascular malformations in infants and children: a classification based on endothelial characteristics. Plast Reconstr Surg 1982;69(3):412–20.
29. Frieden IJ, Haggstrom AN, Drolet BA, et al. Infantile hemangiomas: current knowledge, future directions. proceedings of a research workshop on infantile hemangiomas. Pediatr Dermatol 2005;22(5):383–406.
30. Margileth A, Museles M. Cutaneous hemangiomas in children: diagnosis and conservative management. JAMA 1965;194(5):523–63.
31. North P, Waner M, Mizeracki A, et al. A unique microvascular phenotype shared by juvenile hemangiomas and human placenta. Arch Dermatol 2001;137(5):559–70.
32. Horri K, Drolet B, Frieden I, et al. Prospective study of the frequency of hepatic hemangiomas in infants with multiple cutaneous infantile hemangiomas. Pediatr Dermatol 2011;28(3):245–53.
33. Rosbe K, Suh K, Meyer A, et al. Propanolol management in airway infantile hemangiomas. Arch Otolaryngol Head Neck Surg 2010;136(7):658–65.
34. Leaute-Labreze C, Dumas de la Roque E, Hubiche T, et al. Propanolol for severe hemangiomas of infancy. N Engl J Med 2008;358:2649–51.
35. Drolet B, Frommelt P, Chamlin S, et al. Initiation and use of propranolol for infantile hemangioma: report of a consensus conference. Pediatrics 2013;139(2):153–6.
36. Richter G, Braswell L. Management of venous malformations. Facial Plast Surg 2012;28(6):603–10.
37. Burrows P, Mason K. Percutaneous treatment of low flow vascular malformations. J Vasc Interv Radiol 2004;15(5):431–45.
38. Perkins J, Manning S, Tempero R, et al. Lymphatic malformations: current cellular and clinical investigations. Otolaryngol Head Neck Surg 2010;142(6):789–94.
39. Donaldson SS. Rhabdomyosarcoma: contemporary status and future directions. The Lucy Wortham James Clinical Research Award. Arch Surg 1989;124(9):1015–20.
40. Dagher R, Helman L. Rhabdomyosarcoma: an overview. Oncologist 1999;4(1):34–44.
41. Hennekam RC. Costello syndrome: an overview. Am J Med Genet C Semin Med Genet 2003;117C(1):42–8.
42. Smith AC, Squire JA, Thorner P, et al. Association of alveolar rhabdomyosarcoma with the Beckwith-Wiedemann syndrome. Pediatr Dev Pathol 2001;4(6):550–8.
43. Barr FG. Soft tissue tumors: alveolar rhabdomyosarcoma. Atlas Genet Cytogenet Oncol Haematol 2009;13(12):981–5.
44. Lawrence W Jr, Hays DM, Heyn R, et al. Lymphatic metastases with childhood rhabdomyosarcoma. A report from the Intergroup Rhabdomyosarcoma Study. Cancer 1987;60(4):910–5.

Subglottic Stenosis

Alexander P. Marston, MD, David R. White, MD*

KEYWORDS

- Congenital subglottic stenosis • Acquired subglottic stenosis
- Prolonged endotracheal intubation • Subglottic balloon dilation
- Laryngotracheal reconstruction • Cricotracheal resection

KEY POINTS

- Optimization of endotracheal tube and ventilator management has decreased the rate of acquired subglottic stenosis in neonates with a history of prolonged intubation to as low as 1%.
- Congenital subglottic stenosis is more likely to be associated with a syndrome, whereas acquired subglottic stenosis overwhelmingly occurs in patients with a history of endotracheal intubation.
- Airway management for patients with mild to moderate subglottic stenosis ranges from observation to minimally invasive procedures, such as balloon dilation and endoscopic cricoid split techniques.
- Severe subglottic stenosis often necessitates a tracheostomy to establish a safe and patent airway, with open airway reconstruction considered for patients who are candidates for eventual tracheostomy decannulation.
- Open airway surgical procedures are separated into 3 broad categories: expansion, resection, and slide tracheoplasty techniques.

INTRODUCTION

Neonatal airway stenosis can be congenital or acquired and most commonly occurs within the subglottis. The subglottis is an anatomic region below the level of the vocal folds extending inferiorly to the lower border of the cricoid cartilage. The surrounding structures include the thyroid cartilage and cricothyroid membrane superiorly and the trachea inferiorly. The cricoid is the only complete cartilaginous ring within the airway. As a result, the fixed diameter of this section of the airway makes even subtle edema or scarring a potentially life-threatening airway condition.

Disclosure: No financial disclosure or conflicts of interest to report.
Division of Pediatric Otolaryngology, Department of Otolaryngology–Head and Neck Surgery, MUSC Children's Hospital, Medical University of South Carolina, 135 Rutledge Avenue, MSC 550, Charleston, SC 29425, USA
* Corresponding author.
E-mail address: whitedr@musc.edu

The subglottis is the narrowest section of the airway in infants and young children. A subglottic diameter of 4 mm or less is considered stenotic in a full term neonate, whereas a diameter of 3 mm or less is considered stenotic in a preterm neonate.[1] The severity of subglottic stenosis is determined in a standardized fashion by comparing the appropriate endotracheal tube size with age-matched norms per the Cotton-Myer grading system[2]:

- Grade I: up to 50% stenosis
- Grade II: 51% to 70% stenosis
- Grade III: 71% to 99% stenosis
- Grade IV: no lumen present

Advances in perinatal medicine throughout the twentieth century led to a significant decrease in neonatal intensive care unit mortality; however, this was also associated with an increase in prolonged endotracheal intubation. As a result, the incidence of subglottic stenosis increased at that time. Literature from the 1960s and 1970s reported subglottic stenosis rates ranging between 12% and 20% among neonatal patients requiring prolonged periods of intubation.[3] However, improved medical, ventilator, and endotracheal tube management led to a decrease in adverse events in this population and the subglottic stenosis risk has now stabilized at approximately 1%.[4]

Congenital Subglottic Stenosis

Congenital subglottic stenosis is the third most common congenital anomaly of the airway after laryngomalacia and vocal fold paralysis.[5] It occurs when subglottic patency is narrowed in the absence of prior intubation or airway instrumentation and is commonly observed as a feature of a syndromic diagnosis, such as trisomy 21, CHARGE, and 22q11 deletion syndromes. The cricoid cartilage derives from the sixth branchial arch and forms early in embryologic development.[3] Recanalization of the airway within the cricoid cartilage occurs by the 10th week of gestation and failure of this process leads to subglottic stenosis. Congenital subglottic stenosis can be either membranous or cartilaginous and varies from mild narrowing to complete laryngeal atresia depending on the severity of incomplete cricoid recanalization. A common mild form of congenital cartilaginous subglottic stenosis is observed as an elliptical cricoid with lateral cartilaginous shelves limiting the diameter of the airway (**Fig. 1**).[1] These mild cases of subglottic stenosis often present with persistent stridor or recurrent croup. In the absence of other comorbidities, mild subglottic stenosis can be managed conservatively with symptomatic improvement and greater airway patency as the child grows. In severe cases of congenital subglottic stenosis, abnormal shelves of cartilage fill the inner concave surfaces of the anterolateral cricoid leaving only a small posterior subglottic airway.[6] Such cases represent severe grade III and IV subglottic stenosis and require expeditious surgical management to secure the airway with subsequent reconstructive surgery for appropriately selected patients.

Acquired Subglottic Stenosis

Acquired subglottic stenosis is the most common acquired laryngeal anomaly, with 90% of cases attributable to prior intubation.[7] The current risk of developing subglottic stenosis among neonatal patients intubated for a prolonged period of time is approximately 1%.[4] Anatomic constraints of the subglottis make it susceptible to iatrogenic injury, prolonged healing, and resulting stenosis. Therefore, preventive strategies are important to limit the risk of developing subglottic stenosis.

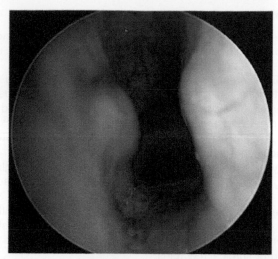

Fig. 1. Direct laryngoscopy view of an elliptical cricoid with lateral cartilaginous shelves. This condition is a common mild form of congenital cartilaginous subglottic stenosis.

Mechanism

The relationship of an inappropriately large endotracheal tube and the development of acquired subglottis stenosis is well established.[3] A large endotracheal tube can cause adjacent pressure necrosis within the subglottis, leading to mucosal edema and ulceration. As the insult progresses, normal mucosal ciliary flow is disrupted, predisposing to infection and perichondritis.[3] The ulcerated subglottic site heals by secondary intention, with deposition of granulation tissue and fibrotic scar resulting in stenosis. Healing of the subglottis is further restricted by a poor blood supply and constant motion of the larynx as a result of head movement and swallowing.[8,9] The resulting transient edema and mature scar lead to significant airway narrowing.

Additional factors that contribute to and increase the risk of developing acquired subglottic stenosis include traumatic intubation, duration of intubation, infection, and gastroesophageal reflux (GER).[10]

Prevention

- Intubation with an appropriately sized endotracheal tube is paramount to minimizing subglottic injury.
- Polymeric silicone and polyvinyl chloride are the safest endotracheal tube materials available.[3]
- An appropriately sized endotracheal tube allows for an air leak between 10 and 30 cm H_2O.[11,12]
- Children with Down syndrome should be intubated with an endotracheal tube 1 full size smaller than the age-appropriate size (eg, 3.5 instead of a 4.5 endotracheal tube) as a result of a smaller airway diameter and higher incidence of congenital subglottic stenosis.[13]
- Maintaining endotracheal tube stability, reducing unexpected extubations and emergent reintubations, and limiting endotracheal tube exchanges are important factors in the prevention of subglottic stenosis.[14,15]
- An experienced perinatal team facilitates optimization of GER treatment, endotracheal tube care, mechanical ventilation, and sedation to limit the risk of developing subglottic stenosis.[3]

Gastroesophageal reflux disease

- GER has the potential to contribute to the development of and/or exacerbate airway conditions, such as chronic cough, stridor,[16] recurrent croup, recurrent pneumonia, and subglottic stenosis.[10]
- Although GER is an important factor in both the work-up and management of subglottic stenosis, it is important to consider that brief episodes of GER occur in approximately 50% of healthy infants less than 2 months old.[17] Once a child reaches 12 months of age, the incidence is estimated at 8%.[18]
- The incidence of GER is reported to be increased in patients with subglottic stenosis, as shown in a report by Walner and colleagues.[10]
  - This study reported that 30% of 74 patients with total subglottic stenosis at an average age of 5 years showed a high risk for GER based on pH probe data.
- Although the association or possible causative effect of GER with subglottic stenosis is not conclusively understood, patients with subglottic stenosis are best managed when their reflux symptoms are optimized by means of conservative, medical, and/or surgical therapies.
- More conclusive evidence is available to support GER optimization before airway reconstruction procedures.
  - Gray and colleagues[19] reported that patients with uncontrolled GER compared with patients without GER have a higher rate of failure following laryngotracheal reconstruction.
  - Therefore, many pediatric otolaryngologists coordinate a thorough GER work-up before performing airway reconstructive procedures.[20]

Sedation management

- Establishing endotracheal tube stability is important because frequent patient movement can lead to ulceration of the delicate subglottic mucosa, followed by fibrinous granulation deposition and subglottic stenosis.
- Schweiger and colleagues[21] published a 2017 study that prospectively investigated the significance of sedation scores in intubated pediatric patients as a possible risk factor for the development of subglottic stenosis.
  - Among 36 patients between the ages of 30 days and 5 years, 4 (11.1%) developed subglottic stenosis.
  - Patients with subglottic stenosis had a higher incidence of undersedation per a standardized sedation assessment compared with patients who did not develop subglottic stenosis (15.8% vs 3.65%, $P = .004$), which suggests that children who went on to develop subglottic stenosis were less sedated than those who did not develop subglottic stenosis.

EVALUATION

Work-up in a patient with possible subglottic stenosis begins with a thorough history and physical examination with an emphasis on excluding nonlaryngeal causes of airway obstruction. Historical factors, such as birth history, prematurity, syndromic diagnoses, congenital anomalies, prior intubations, feeding status, and voice quality, are important to consider. The examination most importantly includes characterization of the patient's respiratory status and endoscopic airway evaluation. Subglottic stenosis most commonly presents in the setting of biphasic stridor. Comparatively, supraglottic abnormalities present with inspiratory stridor and intrathoracic tracheal disorders present with expiratory stridor. Flexible fiberoptic laryngoscopy is performed at the bedside in awake patients in order to evaluate the upper aerodigestive tract, observe the dynamic function of the larynx, and assess for possible laryngomalacia and vocal fold immobility. Depending on the patient's clinical status, examination findings, and level of suspicion for subglottic disorder, a rigid direct laryngoscopy and bronchoscopy under general anesthesia is indicated to formally evaluate the airway distal to the level of the vocal cords.

Airway Endoscopy

Awake flexible fiberoptic laryngoscopy:

- The advantages of awake laryngoscopy include assessment of dynamic airway collapse and vocal cord mobility.
- The disadvantage of this technique is the inability to evaluate distal to the vocal folds in pediatric patients.
- Sinonasal cavity: evaluate for congenital masses, such as nasolacrimal duct cysts and polyps, piriform aperture stenosis, and nasoseptal deviation.
- Nasopharynx: assess for choanal atresia, nasopharyngeal stenosis, and adenoid hypertrophy.
- Oropharynx: evaluate for tonsil hypertrophy; base of tongue obstruction; pharyngomalacia; and masses, such as a vallecular cyst.
- Larynx: assess for laryngomalacia; vocal cord immobility; or an obstructive laryngeal mass, such as a saccular cyst or laryngocele.

Rigid direct laryngoscopy and bronchoscopy:

- Rigid airway endoscopy is performed under general anesthesia and allows thorough investigation of the upper and lower airway structures, including the subglottis, trachea, carina, and bronchial structures.
- A perioperative steroid is administered to minimize edema following airway instrumentation.
- Evaluation of dynamic airway collapse and vocal cord immobility are limited with this technique because of the presence of general anesthesia.
- Subglottis: assess for subglottic stenosis; subglottic cyst; or possible vascular anomaly, such as a subglottic hemangioma.
  - A diagnosis of subglottic stenosis is made by comparing the endotracheal tube size that allows an air leak at less than 30 cm H_2O with age-appropriate endotracheal tube size standards per the Cotton-Myer grading scale.
- Trachea: evaluate for complete tracheal rings; external tracheal compression from adjacent vascular structures, such as in the setting of a vascular ring or aberrant subclavian artery; or an infectious cause such as bacterial tracheitis. Despite the limitations of general anesthesia on dynamic airway collapse evaluation, the examiner can typically assess for the presence or absence of tracheomalacia.

Imaging

- Although endoscopy is the gold standard for subglottic evaluation, adjunct imaging studies may provide further diagnostic information.
- Inspiratory and expiratory plain radiograph films can assess for obstructive bronchial lesions, such as in the case of an aspirated foreign body, and evaluate for pulmonary parenchymal disorder.
- In the setting of subglottic stenosis, anterior-posterior cervical films show a characteristic narrowed appearance known as the steeple sign (**Fig. 2**).

Multispecialty Work-Up

- Patients with subglottic stenosis often have multiple comorbid medical conditions. Therefore, multidisciplinary pediatric subspecialty work-up is often necessary, including genetics, neurology, cardiology, pulmonology, and gastroenterology.
- An understanding of the patient's swallow function and reflux severity are particularly important when considering an airway reconstruction in a patient with subglottic stenosis and tracheostomy dependence.
- For patients with coexisting dysphagia or an aspiration concern, a modified barium swallow study or functional evaluation of swallowing study can provide additional clinical information.

MANAGEMENT

Treatment options for subglottic stenosis have advanced significantly over the past half-century; however, airway stenosis management remains both complex and challenging for pediatric otolaryngologists (**Table 1**). Mild cases of subglottic stenosis (Cotton-Myer grade I and II) can typically be managed conservatively, whereas moderate to severe cases of stenosis (Cotton-Myer grade III and IV) often require surgical intervention and long-term tracheostomy dependence.[3] Although tracheostomy placement may be unavoidable for severe subglottic stenosis, current management techniques, such as endoscopic balloon dilation[22] and laryngotracheoplasty,[23] are targeted at reducing tracheostomy incidence for patients with mild and moderate disease states. Decannulation of the tracheostomy tube can be achieved by means of surgical intervention in medically appropriate patients. Surgical techniques are broadly grouped into either endoscopic or open procedures. Endoscopic procedures, such balloon dilation or endoscopic posterior cricoid split with cartilage graft, are best chosen for patients with isolated subglottic stenosis without a history of prior treatment failure. Open surgical techniques are reserved for more severe grades of subglottic stenosis and patients with multilevel disease. Laryngotracheal reconstruction,[24] cricotracheal resection,[25] and cervical slide tracheoplasty[26] are among the most commonly used open airway reconstruction procedures.

When possible, avoidance of tracheostomy placement is a priority of care because of the high medical and nursing care costs, need for multiple procedures, risk of developing tracheomalacia, tracheostoma bleeding, negative impact on speech

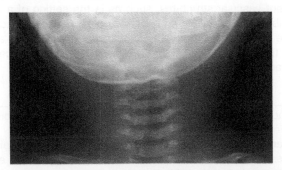

Fig. 2. An anterior-posterior cervical radiograph film shows the characteristic narrowed appearance of the airway in the setting of subglottic stenosis. This finding is referred to as the steeple sign.

Table 1
Subglottic stenosis management

Treatment Modality	Patient and Treatment Factors
Elective period of endotracheal intubation	May be preferred in small neonates; allow for treatment of infection, GER, and inflammation
Endoscopic balloon dilation	Mild to moderate stenosis; acquired disease; soft, immature scar
Endoscopic anterior cricoid split with balloon dilation	Mild to moderate stenosis; repeated failed extubation attempts; failed endoscopic balloon dilation
Endoscopic posterior cricoid split with cartilage graft	Posteriorly based mature subglottic stenosis; posterior glottis stenosis; bilateral vocal cord paralysis
LTR	Grade II or III subglottic stenosis nonresponsive to endoscopic treatments; grade IV stenosis not amenable to CTR
CTR	Severe grade III or IV subglottic stenosis; stenosis extends into trachea; salvage surgery after failed LTR; stenosis must be >3 mm from the vocal folds
Tracheostomy	Need for prolonged mechanical ventilation; multiple medical-comorbidities prohibiting other treatment options; management of severe stenosis until candidate for open reconstruction; unsuccessful previous surgery

Abbreviations: CTR, cricotracheal resection; LTR, laryngotracheal reconstruction.

development, poor voice quality, and 1% to 2% risk of death[1] each year caused by accidental decannulation or obstruction.

Endoscopic Balloon Dilation

Endoscopic balloon dilation is a straightforward, minimally invasive, and effective treatment of appropriately selected patients with subglottic stenosis.[27] Patients with a history of acute acquired subglottic stenosis (diagnosis made ≤30 days following extubation) have immature and soft stenosis and are therefore better candidates for balloon dilation (**Fig. 3**). Comparatively, patients with chronic acquired subglottic stenosis (diagnosis made >30 days following extubation) are less likely to benefit from balloon dilation because of the mature and firm consistency of the stenosis. In addition, balloon dilation is not recommended in patients with congenital subglottic stenosis because of the dense cartilaginous nature of the narrowed airway segment or in long segments of stenosis that extend beyond the subglottis. Balloon dilation is intended to mechanically interrupt the process of scar maturation following an insult to the subglottic airway, such as occurs from prolonged intubation.[22] A unique mechanistic advantage of dilation is that the balloon exerts a radial force over the segment of stenosis, thereby reducing the risk of mucosal injury or airway rupture.[1]

Technique: endoscopic balloon dilation

- Direct laryngoscopy and bronchoscopy are performed in the operating room under general anesthesia.
- The supraglottis, glottis, subglottis, trachea, carina, and bronchi are evaluated and photodocumentation is achieved with a Hopkins rod telescope.
- The subglottic airway is sized per the Cotton-Myer grading system.

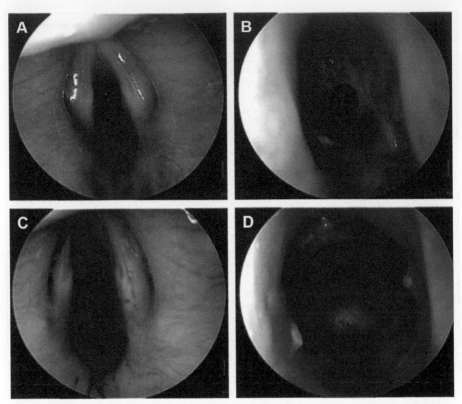

Fig. 3. (*A*, *B*) Direct laryngoscopy reveals a thin, immature, circumferential band of scar tissue consistent with acute acquired subglottic stenosis. (*C*, *D*) Direct laryngoscopy after balloon dilation shows resolution of the subglottic scar band.

- Although variable depending on patient circumstances, the balloon size is typically chosen by adding 2 mm to the outer diameter of the age-appropriate endotracheal tube size for the patient.[28]
- The balloon is placed under visualization with a telescope and inflated to the recommended atmospheric pressure (**Fig. 4**).
- The balloon can remain inflated for up to 2 minutes if tolerated by the patient without significant oxygen desaturation. Repeat dilation can be performed, if deemed appropriate.
- The airway is then resized to objectively assess for improvement gained from the dilation procedure.

Postoperative cares: endoscopic balloon dilation

- Depending on the severity of the subglottic stenosis and how the airway was managed preoperatively, the procedure concludes with a plan to wake the patient up without an endotracheal tube or to return to the intensive care unit with an endotracheal tube in place.
- Neonatal patients are often kept intubated to ensure safe transfer and allow transient postdilation edema to resolve. The intensive care unit administers periextubational steroids for up to 48 hours, with extubation attempted once an air leak

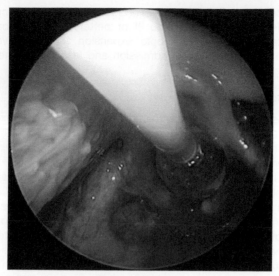

Fig. 4. Endoscopic balloon dilation of the subglottis. The balloon is placed under visualization with a telescope and inflated to the recommended atmospheric pressure.

develops around the endotracheal tube and the ventilator settings are appropriately weaned.

Outcomes: endoscopic balloon dilation

- Endoscopic balloon dilation of the subglottis has reduced the need for open airway reconstruction by an estimated 80%.[29]
- In a prospective study by Avelino and colleagues[28] published in 2015, 48 patients with subglottic stenosis with a mean age of 20.7 months underwent balloon dilation and outcomes were assessed. Ninety-six percent of patients had either grade II or III subglottic stenosis. The success of balloon dilation treatments in patients with acute subglottic stenosis was 100%, whereas in patients with chronic subglottic stenosis the success rate was only 39% ($P<.0001$). In addition, both lower grade of stenosis and younger age were associated with better outcomes.
- A meta-analysis by Lang and Brietzke[27] published in 2014 included 7 studies and 150 pediatric patients with subglottic stenosis treated with balloon dilation. The mean patient age was 2.2 years. Over an average follow-up period of 4.6 months, the random effects model estimate of treatment success was 65.3% (range 50%–100%) with 1.6 mean dilations per patient. Similar to the Avelino and colleagues[28] results, the regression analysis from this article revealed decreased odds of success with increasing severity of stenosis.

In cases of failed endoscopic balloon dilation, Chen and colleagues[30] proposed an endoscopic anterior cricoid split combined with a balloon dilation procedure. This combination can serve as an intermediate alternative for a failed balloon dilation procedure before proceeding with open airway surgery or tracheostomy.

Endoscopic Expansion Surgery

For cases of long-standing subglottic stenosis not amenable to balloon dilation, expansion surgery is necessary to increase the diameter of the subglottic airway. In

2003, Inglis and colleagues[31] described an endoscopic posterior cricoid split with rib graft technique for patients with grade III or better posteriorly based subglottic stenosis. Advantages of an endoscopic expansion technique versus an open approach include a shorter hospital admission and less use of the intensive care unit postoperatively.

Technique: endoscopic expansion surgery

- General anesthesia is induced in the operating room with an existing tracheostomy tube or via endotracheal tube placement.
- A rib graft is harvested from an inframammary incision. Typically, a 2-cm cartilaginous section of the fourth or fifth rib is available.
- Suspension laryngoscopy is performed with a Lindholm laryngoscope supported on a Mayo stand.
  - The plane of anesthesia is managed to allow spontaneous respiration through insufflation of anesthetic gases and intravenous administration of propofol.
- Placement of a vocal cord spreader retracts the vocal cords laterally and allows access to the posterior cricoid plate.
- Laser precautions are instituted. The fraction of inspired oxygen is maintained at less than 30%, wet gauze pads are placed over the eyes, and the patient is covered in wet towels.
- A CO_2 laser system delivered via a flexible fiber allows a precise and hemostatic incision through the posterior cricoid mucosa.
- An endolaryngeal knife, such as a sickle knife, is used to completely incise through the posterior cricoid plate. Care is taken to preserve the posterior aspect of the cricoid perichondrium (**Fig. 5**).
- The optimal graft size is estimated and the cartilage is carved.
  - Approximate graft dimensions are as follows: width of 5 mm, anterior-posterior height of 4 mm, and superior-inferior length of 15 mm.
  - The graft is carved with flanges that will fit deep and lateral to the cut edges of the cricoid plate to allow the graft to snap into place and remain secure.

Postoperative cares: endoscopic expansion surgery

- The airway is stented with either an endotracheal tube or suprastomal stent depending on tracheostomy status for between 1 and 8 weeks.

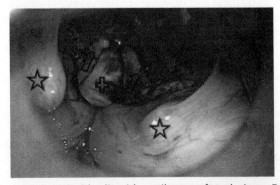

Fig. 5. Endoscopic posterior cricoid split with cartilage graft technique. Endolaryngeal view of a split posterior cricoid cartilage (cut edges labeled with *arrows*) with preserved deep cricoid perichondrium (labeled with a *plus sign*). The arytenoids are labeled with stars.

○ If an endotracheal tube is maintained, the patient is kept under an appropriate level of sedation in the intensive care unit to minimize movement and ensure stability of the airway.

- Before extubation or removal of the tracheostomy tube, repeat airway examination is completed to ensure that the graft remains in the desired position and is mucosalized with minimal airway edema/granulation tissue.

Outcomes: endoscopic expansion surgery

- A 2017 publication by Dahl and colleagues[32] summarized their cumulative endoscopic posterior cricoid split with rib graft results:
  ○ Thirteen patients with subglottic stenosis and tracheostomy dependence underwent an endoscopic posterior cricoid cartilage split with rib graft placement at a mean age of 4.15 years.
  ○ Decannulation was achieved in 53.8% of patients following the endoscopic rib graft procedure and hence did not require an open airway surgical intervention.
- Most cases of subglottic stenosis involve some degree of circumferential narrowing and are, therefore, less likely to benefit from an endoscopic posterior cartilage graft. Nevertheless, this technique offers a less invasive surgery for a select group of patients with mild to moderate posteriorly based subglottic stenosis.

Open Airway Reconstruction

Open airway surgical procedures are categorized into 3 general classifications:

1. Expansion surgery
2. Resection surgery
3. Slide tracheoplasty

Patients with moderate to severe subglottic stenosis (**Fig. 6**) or multilevel airway obstruction are more likely to achieve successful outcomes from open, rather than endoscopic, surgical techniques.[33] Although open airway surgery carries a higher risk of morbidity, this is counteracted by it allowing a definitive airway intervention. Open airway surgical morbidity includes, but is not limited to, longer hospitalization, neck scarring, worse voice quality, and potentially compromised swallow outcomes.[3] Nevertheless, a single open operation for patients with moderate to severe subglottic stenosis is preferred rather than multiple, perhaps futile, endoscopic procedures. It is critical to consider that the best chance for a successful airway intervention is at the time of the primary surgical procedure.[34] Therefore, avoidance of multiple inappropriately selected airway surgeries is paramount.

Laryngotracheal Reconstruction

Laryngotracheal reconstruction is often most appropriate for patients with complex or refractory grade II and grade III subglottic stenosis. The severity and location of the airway disease dictates the type of expansion that will best improve airway patency.[3] For patients with either isolated anterior or isolated posterior subglottic stenosis, an anterior cricoid split with cartilage graft or posterior cricoid split with cartilage graft,[35] respectively, may be the only necessary intervention. In patients with more severe circumferential subglottic stenosis, a combined anterior and posterior cricoid split with cartilage graft placement may be the best reconstructive option.[35]

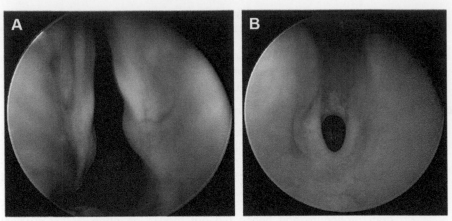

Fig. 6. Direct laryngoscopy evaluation of a patient with chronic acquired grade III subglottic stenosis. (*A*) The glottis and subglottis. (*B*) Zoomed-in view of the subglottis. The stenosis is mature and was not responsive to endoscopic balloon dilation.

Preoperative work-up: laryngotracheal reconstruction

- Infection with methicillin-resistant *Staphylococcus aureus* (MRSA) and *Pseudomonas aeruginosa* is known to increase the complications, failure rate, and mortality following laryngotracheal reconstruction.[36,37]
- Therefore, it is recommended that patients be screened, and treated if positive, for MRSA and pseudomonal infections before laryngotracheal reconstruction.[36,38]

Cartilage grafting material: laryngotracheal reconstruction

- Autologous rib cartilage is the most commonly used grafting material.
  - Advantages:
    - Ability to be carved into a customized size and shape
    - Can be used for either an anterior or posterior cricoid split graft
  - Disadvantages:
    - Requires a separate incision
    - Risk of pneumothorax
- For selected patients, a thyroid ala graft is used
  - Advantage:
    - Easy to harvest via the same cervical incision as the laryngotracheal reconstruction
  - Disadvantages:
    - Provides a limited amount of grafting material
    - Difficult to carve
    - Cannot be used as a posterior cricoid split graft

Single-stage versus double-stage laryngotracheal reconstruction

Laryngotracheal reconstruction can be performed in either a single-stage or double-stage fashion. For patients who are already tracheostomy dependent, single-stage surgery allows for tracheostomy decannulation at the time of the laryngotracheal reconstruction. However, the immediately reconstructed and decannulated airway requires a period of stenting, which is accomplished with maintenance of an endotracheal tube within the airway for between 5 and 10 days. Single-stage reconstructions are best reserved for patients who are undergoing a primary airway reconstruction for isolated subglottic stenosis, can easily be reintubated, and have stable pulmonary function.[39]

A double-stage laryngotracheoplasty procedure maintains the tracheostomy tube during a period of convalescence following the reconstructive surgery. It is appropriate for patients who have failed prior airway reconstruction attempts, have multilevel obstruction, a history of difficult intubation, neurologic deficits, or significant pulmonary disease.[40–42] These circumstances and comorbid conditions are best managed by maintaining a stable tracheostomy airway during the postoperative period. The advantages of the double-stable stage technique include less postoperative sedation, a shorter intensive care unit stay, and elimination of a possible emergent reintubation.

Postoperative airway stenting: laryngotracheal reconstruction

- Following a double-stage laryngotracheoplasty, a suprastomal stent is maintained to preserve the cartilage graft position and reinforce the reconstructed airway.[43]
- Smith and colleagues[44] published a report comparing outcomes for short-term (≤21 days) versus long-term (>21 days) stents in 36 children after laryngotracheoplasty. Decannulation was achieved in 73% of the long-term stent patients but only 36% of the short-term stent patients. When the analysis was adjusted for stenosis grade and age, the long-term stent patients had 4.3 greater odds (95% confidence interval, 1.0–18.3) of decannulation.

Outcomes: single-stage laryngotracheal reconstruction

- In a review of 200 single-stage laryngotracheal reconstructions, Gustafson and colleagues[40] reported an overall decannulation rate of 96%.
  - Twenty-nine percent of patients required reintubation and 15% required a postoperative tracheostomy.
  - Patient age less than 4 years, the placement of both anterior and posterior cartilage grafts, sedation for greater than 48 hours postoperatively, and moderate or severe tracheomalacia all significantly increased the rate of reintubation.

Outcomes: double-stage laryngotracheal reconstruction

- Historically, patients selected for double-stage compared with single-stage airway reconstruction had more severe disease based on grade of subglottic stenosis and vocal cord function.[45,46]
  - Therefore, decreased overall decannulation rates in double-stage compared with single-stage procedures are consistent with more severe and complex airway disease at baseline in the double-stage group.[41,46]
  - Saunders and colleagues[41] published a study in 1999 that described an overall decannulation rate of 91.4% in the single-stage group versus 61.8% in the double-stage group.
- A more recent study by Smith and colleagues[39] published in 2010 showed similar double-stage and single-stage overall decannulation rates.
  - Eighty-four laryngotracheal reconstructions (22 single stage and 62 double stage) from a single institution were reviewed retrospectively.
  - The mean grade of subglottic stenosis per the Cotton-Myer grading scale was 2.1 in the single-stage group and 2.9 in the double-stage group.
  - Overall decannulation rates were not significantly different between the single-stage (100%) and the double-stage (93%) groups despite worse disease severity in the double-stage cohort.

o Advances in the technical aspects of the double-stage procedure were postulated to allow comparable double-stage and single-stage decannulation rates:
  ▪ Placement of the posterior cricoid split graft without sutures
  ▪ Shorter postoperative stenting time

CRICOTRACHEAL RESECTION

Cricotracheal resection is indicated for severe grade 3 and 4 subglottic stenosis or in patients with an insufficient subglottis and history of failed laryngotracheal reconstruction. Although laryngotracheal reconstruction expands open a stenotic subglottic airway by means of inserting cartilage grafts within a split cricoid cartilage, a cricotracheal resection addresses the problem by excising the narrowed subglottic airway segment. The technique should not be used when the stenosis is within 3 mm of the vocal cords; with very long segment stenosis; or if mobilization of the distal trachea is difficult, such as in the setting of prior tracheoesophageal fistula repair.

In this procedure, the anterior aspect of the cricoid cartilage is removed, the proximal tracheal stenosis is resected, the posterior half of the cricoid plate is thinned with a drill, and the trachea is advanced superiorly to be anastomosed with the thyroid cartilage anteriorly and the remaining cricoid cartilage posteriorly.

Outcomes: Cricotracheal Resection

- Decannulation rates for cricotracheal resection are reported to exceed 90%.[25]
- White and colleagues[25] reported on their institutional experience of 93 consecutive cricotracheal resections and found an overall decannulation rate of 94% and an operation-specific decannulation rate of 71%.[2]
  o The overall decannulation rate included patients who were decannulated after the cricotracheal resection, as well as patients who required a cricotracheal resection plus additional airway surgical interventions.
  o This study found that unilateral and bilateral vocal fold paralysis were significant risk factors for failure to decannulate after cricotracheal resection.

Cervical Slide Tracheoplasty

Slide tracheoplasty surgery was originally designed to treat isolated tracheal stenosis, such as in patients with complete tracheal rings. However, this procedure can be applied to patients with combined subglottic and tracheal stenosis by incorporating the anterior aspect of the cricoid ring within the slide tracheoplasty technique.[26] This procedure can be accomplished via either a transcervical or transthoracic approach depending on the surgical access needed.

SUMMARY

The subglottis is a narrow and delicate site within the pediatric airway that is exquisitely susceptible to the development of airway stenosis. Contributing factors to the sensitivity of the subglottis include the presence of friable mucosa, limited blood supply, and the inability of this segment of the airway to expand. The incidence of acquired subglottic stenosis in the setting of prolonged intubation has significantly decreased as a result of improved endotracheal tube and ventilator management and optimized sedation protocols. Thorough evaluation of the airway is recommended when subglottic stenosis is suspected to both rule out coexisting airway abnormalities and characterize the severity and extent of subglottic disorder. Advances in otolaryngology surgical procedures, such as endoscopic balloon dilation and endoscopic cricoid split with cartilage graft techniques, allow minimally invasive treatment options and possible avoidance of tracheostomy for patients with mild to moderate subglottic stenosis. However, patients with severe subglottic stenosis, failed primary surgery, additional sites of airway obstruction, and/or comorbid conditions are often tracheostomy dependent. Open surgical techniques to definitively treat severe subglottic stenosis, such as laryngotracheal reconstruction and cricotracheal resection, offer a high rate of symptom resolution and eventual tracheostomy decannulation.

Best Practices

What is the current practice?

Ensure a safe and stable airway in patients with subglottic stenosis. For patients with severe subglottic stenosis, tracheostomy or airway reconstruction is necessary to establish a viable airway.

Best practice/guideline/care path objective

The risk of developing subglottic stenosis is minimized in intubated neonates through careful sedation management, optimization of ventilator settings, minimizing endotracheal tube movement, and eliminating unnecessary endotracheal tube exchanges.

What changes in practice are likely to improve outcomes?

Future advances in endoscopic airway techniques and instrumentation will allow more precise treatment and further avoid the need to perform open surgical airway procedures.

Is there a clinical algorithm?

There is no single clinical algorithm as a result of the heterogeneity in type and severity of subglottic stenosis. **Table 1** provides a general overview of the selection of appropriate surgical intervention.

Clinical algorithm

- Immature, mild severity subglottic stenosis can be treated initially with endoscopic balloon dilation.
- Mature, moderate to severe subglottic stenosis is unlikely to improve from dilation techniques and requires either endoscopic or open reconstructive airway surgery.

Major recommendations

- Work closely with the neonatal intensive care unit to ensure that endotracheal tube management is optimized to reduce the risk of acquired subglottic stenosis.
- Confirm adequate pulmonary function, minimal oxygen supplementation, and no mechanical ventilation needs before airway reconstruction.
- Carefully select the timing and type of surgical procedure because the primary intervention has the highest chance of success.[34]

Rating for the strength of evidence

The strength of evidence classification for the analysis provided in this article is B. Although ample literature is available and numerous high-volume series have been reported, few randomized studies exist.

Bibliographic source

The clinical experience of the authors and published literature were used to describe the recommendations presented in this article.

Summary statement

Subglottic stenosis is a challenging condition that can present as a congenital or acquired lesion and range in severity from mild, asymptomatic stenosis to severe stenosis and tracheostomy dependence. Collaboration with multidisciplinary pediatric subspecialty teams and careful surgical decision making are critical in selecting the best treatment options for these patients.

REFERENCES

1. Jefferson ND, Cohen AP, Rutter MJ. Subglottic stenosis. Semin Pediatr Surg 2016;25(3):138–43.
2. Myer CM 3rd, O'Connor DM, Cotton RT. Proposed grading system for subglottic stenosis based on endotracheal tube sizes. Ann Otol Rhinol Laryngol 1994;103(4 Pt 1):319–23.
3. Lesperance MM, Flint PW. Cummings pediatric otolaryngology. Philadelphia: Elsevier/Saunders; 2015.
4. Choi SS, Zalzal GH. Changing trends in neonatal subglottic stenosis. Otolaryngol Head Neck Surg 2000;122(1):61–3.
5. Rutter MJ. Congenital laryngeal anomalies. Braz J Otorhinolaryngol 2014;80(6): 533–9.
6. Cotton R. Management of subglottic stenosis in infancy and childhood. Review of a consecutive series of cases managed by surgical reconstruction. Ann Otol Rhinol Laryngol 1978;87(5 Pt 1):649–57.
7. Rodriguez H, Cuestas G, Botto H, et al. Post-intubation subglottic stenosis in children. Diagnosis, treatment and prevention of moderate and severe stenosis. Acta Otorrinolaringol Esp 2013;64(5):339–44.
8. Gould SJ, Young M. Subglottic ulceration and healing following endotracheal intubation in the neonate: a morphometric study. Ann Otol Rhinol Laryngol 1992;101(10):815–20.
9. Healy GB. An experimental model for the endoscopic correction of subglottic stenosis with clinical applications. Laryngoscope 1982;92(10 Pt 1):1103–15.
10. Walner DL, Stern Y, Gerber ME, et al. Gastroesophageal reflux in patients with subglottic stenosis. Arch Otolaryngol Head Neck Surg 1998;124(5):551–5.
11. Finholt DA, Audenaert SM, Stirt JA, et al. Endotracheal tube leak pressure and tracheal lumen size in swine. Anesth Analg 1986;65(6):667–71.
12. Finholt DA, Henry DB, Raphaely RC. Factors affecting leak around tracheal tubes in children. Can Anaesth Soc J 1985;32(4):326–9.
13. Shott SR. Down syndrome: analysis of airway size and a guide for appropriate intubation. Laryngoscope 2000;110(4):585–92.
14. Jones R, Bodnar A, Roan Y, et al. Subglottic stenosis in newborn intensive care unit graduates. Am J Dis Child 1981;135(4):367–8.
15. Hawkins DB. Pathogenesis of subglottic stenosis from endotracheal intubation. Ann Otol Rhinol Laryngol 1987;96(1 Pt 1):116–7.
16. Orenstein SR, Orenstein DM, Whitington PF. Gastroesophageal reflux causing stridor. Chest 1983;84(3):301–2.
17. Boyle JT. Gastroesophageal reflux in the pediatric patient. Gastroenterol Clin North Am 1989;18(2):315–37.
18. Vandenplas Y, Goyvaerts H, Helven R, et al. Gastroesophageal reflux, as measured by 24-hour pH monitoring, in 509 healthy infants screened for risk of sudden infant death syndrome. Pediatrics 1991;88(4):834–40.
19. Gray S, Miller R, Myer CM 3rd, et al. Adjunctive measures for successful laryngotracheal reconstruction. Ann Otol Rhinol Laryngol 1987;96(5):509–13.
20. Cotton RT, O'Connor DM. Paediatric laryngotracheal reconstruction: 20 years' experience. Acta Otorhinolaryngol Belg 1995;49(4):367–72.
21. Schweiger C, Manica D, Pereira DRR, et al. Undersedation is a risk factor for the development of subglottic stenosis in intubated children. J Pediatr (Rio J) 2017; 93(4):351–5.

22. Durden F, Sobol SE. Balloon laryngoplasty as a primary treatment for subglottic stenosis. Arch Otolaryngol Head Neck Surg 2007;133(8):772–5.
23. Luft JD, Wetmore RF, Tom LW, et al. Laryngotracheoplasty in the management of subglottic stenosis. Int J Pediatr Otorhinolaryngol 1989;17(3):297–303.
24. Cotton RT, Evans JN. Laryngotracheal reconstruction in children. Five-year follow-up. Ann Otol Rhinol Laryngol 1981;90(5 Pt 1):516–20.
25. White DR, Cotton RT, Bean JA, et al. Pediatric cricotracheal resection: surgical outcomes and risk factor analysis. Arch Otolaryngol Head Neck Surg 2005; 131(10):896–9.
26. de Alarcon A, Rutter MJ. Cervical slide tracheoplasty. Arch Otolaryngol Head Neck Surg 2012;138(9):812–6.
27. Lang M, Brietzke SE. A systematic review and meta-analysis of endoscopic balloon dilation of pediatric subglottic stenosis. Otolaryngol Head Neck Surg 2014;150(2):174–9.
28. Avelino M, Maunsell R, Jube Wastowski I. Predicting outcomes of balloon laryngoplasty in children with subglottic stenosis. Int J Pediatr Otorhinolaryngol 2015; 79(4):532–6.
29. Hautefort C, Teissier N, Viala P, et al. Balloon dilation laryngoplasty for subglottic stenosis in children: eight years' experience. Arch Otolaryngol Head Neck Surg 2012;138(3):235–40.
30. Chen C, Ni WH, Tian TL, et al. The outcomes of endoscopic management in young children with subglottic stenosis. Int J Pediatr Otorhinolaryngol 2017;99: 141–5.
31. Inglis AF Jr, Perkins JA, Manning SC, et al. Endoscopic posterior cricoid split and rib grafting in 10 children. Laryngoscope 2003;113(11):2004–9.
32. Dahl JP, Purcell PL, Parikh SR, et al. Endoscopic posterior cricoid split with costal cartilage graft: a fifteen-year experience. Laryngoscope 2017;127(1):252–7.
33. Maresh A, Preciado DA, O'Connell AP, et al. A comparative analysis of open surgery vs endoscopic balloon dilation for pediatric subglottic stenosis. JAMA Otolaryngol Head Neck Surg 2014;140(10):901–5.
34. Bailey M, Hoeve H, Monnier P. Paediatric laryngotracheal stenosis: a consensus paper from three European centres. Eur Arch Otorhinolaryngol 2003;260(3): 118–23.
35. Rizzi MD, Thorne MC, Zur KB, et al. Laryngotracheal reconstruction with posterior costal cartilage grafts: outcomes at a single institution. Otolaryngol Head Neck Surg 2009;140(3):348–53.
36. Ludemann JP, Hughes CA, Noah Z, et al. Complications of pediatric laryngotracheal reconstruction: prevention strategies. Ann Otol Rhinol Laryngol 1999; 108(11 Pt 1):1019–26.
37. Song X, Perencevich E, Campos J, et al. Clinical and economic impact of methicillin-resistant Staphylococcus aureus colonization or infection on neonates in intensive care units. Infect Control Hosp Epidemiol 2010;31(2):177–82.
38. Statham MM, de Alarcon A, Germann JN, et al. Screening and treatment of methicillin-resistant Staphylococcus aureus in children undergoing open airway surgery. Arch Otolaryngol Head Neck Surg 2012;138(2):153–7.
39. Smith LP, Zur KB, Jacobs IN. Single- vs double-stage laryngotracheal reconstruction. Arch Otolaryngol Head Neck Surg 2010;136(1):60–5.
40. Gustafson LM, Hartley BE, Liu JH, et al. Single-stage laryngotracheal reconstruction in children: a review of 200 cases. Otolaryngol Head Neck Surg 2000;123(4): 430–4.

41. Saunders MW, Thirlwall A, Jacob A, et al. Single-or-two-stage laryngotracheal reconstruction; comparison of outcomes. Int J Pediatr Otorhinolaryngol 1999; 50(1):51–4.
42. Boardman SJ, Albert DM. Single-stage and multistage pediatric laryngotracheal reconstruction. Otolaryngol Clin North Am 2008;41(5):947–58, ix.
43. Preciado D. A randomized study of suprastomal stents in laryngotracheoplasty surgery for grade III subglottic stenosis in children. Laryngoscope 2014;124(1): 207–13.
44. Smith DF, de Alarcon A, Jefferson ND, et al. Short- versus long-term stenting in children with subglottic stenosis undergoing laryngotracheal reconstruction. Otolaryngol Head Neck Surg 2018;158(2):375–80.
45. Agrawal N, Black M, Morrison G. Ten-year review of laryngotracheal reconstruction for paediatric airway stenosis. Int J Pediatr Otorhinolaryngol 2007;71(5): 699–703.
46. Hartnick CJ, Hartley BE, Lacy PD, et al. Surgery for pediatric subglottic stenosis: disease-specific outcomes. Ann Otol Rhinol Laryngol 2001;110(12):1109–13.

Neonatal Tracheostomy

Jonathan Walsh, MD[a],*, Jeffrey Rastatter, MD[b]

KEYWORDS

- Tracheostomy • Neonatal • Tracheotomy • Surgical technique • Morbidity
- Outcomes

KEY POINTS

- Cardiopulmonary and neurologic disorders are the primary indications for neonatal tracheostomy.
- A vertical tracheostomy incision with retraction sutures is the predominating surgical technique.
- Neonatal tracheostomy is associated with high overall mortality and morbidity.
- Postoperative and long-term care is needed to help mitigate and manage the increased risks.
- There should be increased awareness of the neurodevelopmental impact associated with tracheostomies in all domains of development.

INTRODUCTION

Neonatal and infant tracheostomy has been a valuable aspect of the care and survival of children over the past century. With the implementation of neonatal and pediatric intensive care units (ICUs), more infants are surviving conditions that in decades past were considered fatal. Tracheostomy plays a vital role in many of these conditions. Although little has changed with regard to technique, there have been significant evolutions in indications, survival, complications, and technological advances.

History

Early tracheotomies were described as far back as 3600 BC. Ancient Egyptian, Greek, and Hindi cultures all reference tracheotomy. Asclepiades is the first referenced individual to perform a tracheotomy around 100 BC. It was not until 1620 when Habicot performed the first pediatric tracheotomy on a 16-year-old boy.[1] In the first half of the 1900s, there were great advances in neonatal resuscitation and ventilation. In 1953, Donald and Lord[2] described a rudimentary infant mechanical ventilation device. In 1965, Mcdonald and Stocks[3] reported prolonged intubation and ventilation in

Disclosure Statement: The authors have no disclosures of any relationship with a commercial company that has a direct financial interest in subject matter or materials discussed in article or with a company making a competing product.
^a Department of Otolaryngology Head and Neck Surgery, Johns Hopkins School of Medicine, 601 North Caroline Street, 6th Floor, Baltimore, MD 21287, USA; ^b Ann & Robert H. Lurie Children's Hospital of Chicago, Box 25, 225 E Chicago Avenue, Chicago, IL 60611, USA
* Corresponding author.
E-mail address: Jwalsh31@jhmi.edu

neonates. In 1971, the concept of continuous positive pressure ventilation for respiratory distress of newborns was published.[4] These advances in neonatal care created new indications for tracheotomy, including postintubation subglottic stenosis and chronic lung disease with prolonged ventilation.

Neonatal Airway Anatomy

The infant and neonatal airway diameter and length vary by gestational age. The narrowest portion of the infant airway is at the glottis and subglottis. This correlates with these sites being the most common locations of postintubation stenosis. In a newborn, the subglottis inner diameter (ID) is 3.5 to 4 mm. The tracheal length from glottis to carina is about 40 mm. Premature infants may have a subglottic airway of less than 3 mm.[5]

Indications or Contraindications

Common indications for tracheostomy are the need for prolonged ventilation, facilitation of ventilator weaning, upper airway obstruction, or infectious causes.[6–17] Over the recent decades, there have been shifts in the most common indications. In recent years, several retrospective studies have demonstrated dramatic drops in infectious causes of tracheostomy and increases in cardiopulmonary and neurologic indications.[8,9,15,17]

Highly unstable pulmonary hypertension or cardiopulmonary disease can be relative contraindications.[16] There are no universally agreed on contraindications for maximum fraction of inspired oxygen (Fi02) levels or peak airway pressure (PAP) levels. A survey of 150 practicing pediatric otolaryngologists found that Fi02 and PAP were not influential in tracheostomy decision.[16] If the neonate is unable to safely be transported to the operating room, be manipulated and positioned for surgery, tolerate exchange of the endotracheal tube to a tracheostomy tube, or if short-term survival is in question, then surgery should be deferred.

There is no absolute weight requirement for tracheostomy procedure.[9–11] However, a limiting factor is the size of the neonatal airway in relation to the smallest available tracheostomy tube outer diameter (OD). A weight of 2 kg is a typical cutoff for when a tracheostomy is placed; however, safe tracheostomy in ultralow-birthweight infants less than 2 kg has been performed. The ID of a full-term newborn is approximately 3.5 to 4 mm. Ultralow-birthweight premature infants may have an ID of 2 mm. The smallest OD tracheostomy tubes are the NEO Bivona 2.5 TTS (Dublin, OH), with an OD of 4.0 mm, and the NEO Shiley Cuffless 2.5 (Medtronic, Minneapolis, MN), with an OD of 4.2 mm. Tracheal length also may be factor in being able to accommodate the standard 30 mm of length of the tracheostomy tubes. Custom tracheostomy tubes can be made to accommodate nonstandard anatomy requirements.

An additional factor in timing and choice of tracheostomy is the innovation and increasing use of noninvasive positive pressure ventilation of newborns. High-flow nasal cannula, nasal SiPAP (synchronized inspiratory positive airway pressure), or continuous positive airway pressure (CPAP) ventilator have enabled prolonged ventilation without intubation. Systematic reviews have demonstrated the efficacy and safety of these methods when compared with traditional orotracheal intubation.[18–20] With possibly fewer intubations, the indications for tracheostomy due to acquired stenosis may be decreasing (**Table 1**).

SURGICAL TECHNIQUE OR PROCEDURE
Preoperative Planning

Due to the often complex and critical nature of neonates who require a tracheostomy, preoperative planning is crucial. As the indications for neonatal tracheostomy vary, so

Table 1
Common indications and contraindications for tracheostomy

Indications	Contraindications
Cardiopulmonary disease, requiring longer term positive pressure ventilation	Critically ill, unable to tolerate anesthesia
Neurologic disorders, congenital and acquired	Critical tracheal stenosis or agenesis
Craniofacial disorders with upper airway obstruction	Craniofacial and cervical dysmorphia that prevents surgical access
Acquired or congenital glottic, subglottic, or tracheal stenosis	Critical cardiac disease necessitating thoracotomy
Congenital high airway obstruction syndrome (CHAOS)[a]	Weight (no absolute cutoff)
Acute airway infections (epiglottitis, tracheitis, croup)	High ventilator settings (no absolute cutoff)

[a] Via the ex utero intrapartum treatment (EXIT) procedure.

does the type of workup and planning required. Coordination and planning with the neonatologists, pulmonologists, cardiologist, and surgeons, as well as the family, is of utmost importance. Not only is identifying whether an infant would benefit from a tracheostomy important but also the timing of tracheostomy with optimization of the clinical condition and coordination with other procedures is often needed.

Medical workup and evaluation may include a complete blood count, coagulation studies, echocardiogram, and chest radiograph. Other questions that may affect the timing and coordination of the procedure are: Will the infant need any cardiac interventions or procedures? Will the infant need a gastrostomy tube? Are there neurologic procedures or interventions needed? What is the primary indication for the tracheotomy and is there expectation that this cause is reversible or expected to improve?

In addition to care coordination, early family integration in the decision, planning, and timing of the tracheostomy is critical because the long-term implications of a neonatal tracheostomy on family care and discharge planning cannot be understated. Family education, teaching, and tracheostomy care skills are important in the success and safety of neonatal tracheotomies. Teaching routine and emergency care, as well as assisting with guiding expectations early, often before the surgery is performed, can help prepare the families.[21,22] Dedicated tracheostomy teaching and education programs can greatly facilitate this process with the use of printed instructional manuals, online resources, high-fidelity simulation training, support groups, and early engagement of families in tracheostomy care. Hospitals may allow for parents to stay in the room to increase comfort and training opportunities, or allow for short trips out of the hospital to increase comfort level before discharge. Community and family support is essential. Resources such as tracheostomy.com provide access to educational materials and support groups.[21,22] Exact requirements of home care varies by location, including the amount of home nursing and number of trained caregivers in the household; however, regardless of legal requirements, training and education should be maximized.

Neonatal tracheostomy tube choices vary by diameter size and length (**Table 2**). Primary manufacturers in the United States are Bivona and Shiley (**Figs. 1–3**).

When choosing a tracheostomy tube, the following decisions must be made:

1. Ensure that the appropriate sizes for the infant's weight are available. Additionally, having 1 size smaller and 1 size larger allows for adaptation to intraoperative

Table 2
Neonatal tracheostomy tube choices: size and length

Tracheostomy Tube		ID (mm)	OD (mm)	Distal Length (mm)	Cuff Option	Material
Bivona (NEO)	2.5	2.5	4	30	Y (TTS)	Silicone
	3	3	4.7	32	Y	Silicone
	3.5	3.5	5.3	34	Y	Silicone
	4	4	6	36	Y	Silicone
Bivona (PED)	2.5	2.5	4	38	Y	Silicone
	3	3	4.7	49	Y	Silicone
	3.5	3.5	5.3	40	Y	Silicone
	4	4	6	41	Y	Silicone
Shiley (NEO)	2.5 NEF	2.5	4.2	30	Y (NCF)	PVC
	3 NEF	3	4.8	30	Y	PVC
	3.5 NEF	3.5	5.4	32	Y	PVC
	4 NEF	4	6.0	34	Y	PVC
	4.5 NEF	4.5	6.7	36	Y	PVC
Shiley (PED)	2.5 PEF	2.5	4.2	39	Y	PVC
	3PEF	3	4.8	39	Y	PVC
	3.5 PEF	4.5	5.4	40	Y	PVC
	4 PEF	4	6.0	41	Y	PVC
	4.5 PEF	4.5	6.5	42	Y	PVC

Abbreviation: PVC, polyvinyl chloride.

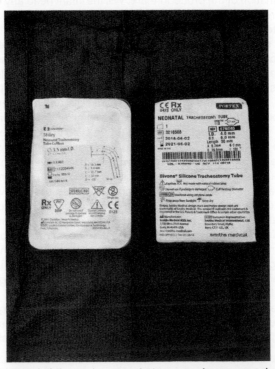

Fig. 1. Standard neonatal Shiley and neonatal Bivona tracheostomy tubes.

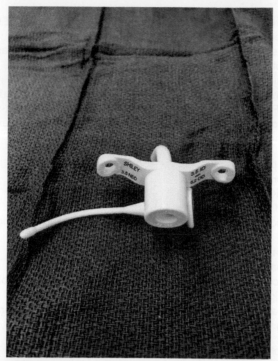

Fig. 2. Neonatal Cuffless Shiley tracheostomy tube with insertion obturator.

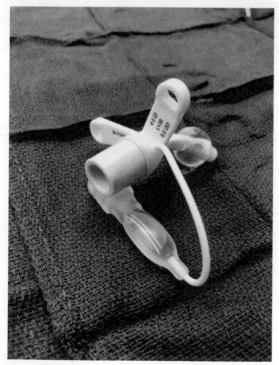

Fig. 3. Neonatal Bivona tight to shaft cuffed tracheostomy tube.

findings. For most infants who are 2 kg or larger, a 3.5 uncuffed NEO Shiley or a 3.0 TTS NEO Bivona is appropriate.

2. Determine whether a cuffed or uncuffed tracheostomy tube is needed. The choice can depend on surgeon preference, hospital tracheostomy tube availability, and the need for high peak pressure ventilation.
3. Determine whether a NEO (neonatal), PED (pediatric), or custom length is needed. The PED length may be needed to accommodate long-segment stenosis or tracheomalacia; however, many neonates may not have the tracheal length necessary for the PED length.

Preparation and patient positioning
- Place a shoulder roll
- Extend neck
- Palpate and mark landmarks
  ○ Sternal notch (feel for great vessel pulsations and high-riding innominate artery)
  ○ Cricoid cartilage
  ○ Thyroid cartilage
- Mark a 1.5 cm horizontal or vertical incision just below the cricoid in the midline, typically 1 figure breadth above the sternal notch
- Inject local anesthesia (0.5% lidocaine with 1:100,000 epinephrine)
- Preparation with betadine.

Surgical approach
Use a horizontal or vertical skin incision.

Surgical procedure
Step 1: Using a 15-blade scalpel, make a 1.5 cm skin incision just inferior to the cricoid cartilage and 1 finger breadth above the sternal notch.
Step 2: Excise the subcutaneous fat to expose the cervical fascia and strap muscles.
Step 3: Identify the midline raphe and separate the strap muscles vertically (neonatal anatomy can be difficult to identify and palpate makes it easy to inadvertently extend the dissection lateral to the trachea; care must be taken to remain in the midline).
Step 4: The strap muscles are retracted laterally with small vein retractors or Senn retractors.
Step 5: Identify the cricoid cartilage and thyroid isthmus.
Step 6: Isolate the thyroid isthmus with a small dissecting clamp and divide with bipolar cautery.
Step 7: Identify the tracheal rings 2 through 4.
Step 8: Deflate the endotracheal tube cuff (to avoid inadvertent cuff puncture) and place tracheal retraction sutures through 2 tracheal rings oriented vertically with 3-0 Prolene (Ethicon, Somerville, NJ) sutures.
Step 9: (optional) Using 5-0 chromic sutures, tack the skin edges to the superior and inferior edges of the trachea to mature the stoma.[23]
Step 10: Using a 15-blade scalpel, make a vertical incision through tracheal rings 2 through 4 in the midline between the 2 retraction sutures (**Fig. 4**).
Step 11: Carefully pull back the endotracheal tube until the tip is just above the tracheostomy incision.
Step 12: Place an appropriately sized tracheostomy tube into the tracheostomy incision.

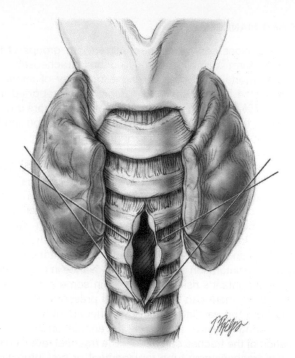

Fig. 4. Vertical incision through tracheal rings. (Tim Phelps © JHU 2018/AAM. Department of Art as Applied to Medicine. Johns Hopkins University School of Medicine.)

Step 13: Confirm placement with return of end-tidal carbon dioxide, appropriate tidal volumes, and/or passing a suction catheter easily.

Step 14: Using a small fiberoptic laryngoscope through the tracheotomy tube, confirm that the distal tip of the tracheostomy tube is the appropriate length above the carina.

Step 15: Place tracheostomy tube ties and secure the tube.

Step 16: (optional) Consider placing skin-protecting dressing (DuoDERM [Bridgewater, NJ], Mepilex [Gothenburg, Sweden]) to limit skin breakdown during the healing process. The neck, chin, and chest are common sites of skin pressure ulceration.

Step 17: Label each Prolene retraction suture as left or right, as appropriate, and tape to the chest. These sutures are pulled in their anatomic direction in the event of a decannulation to assist with tracheostomy tube replacement, or they can be pulled in the opposite direction to assist with orotracheal intubation if tracheostomy tube replacement is unsuccessful.

Step 18: When the tracheostomy is secured and confirmed to be functioning for adequate ventilation, remove the oral endotracheal tube.

ALTERNATE TECHNIQUE (STARPLASTY)

The starplasty technique uses the principles of a Z-plasty to create a stomatized tracheostomy. A cruciate skin incision is made 1 cm by 1 cm.[24,25] The subcutaneous fat is removed and the strap muscles and thyroid gland are divided. Next, a cruciate tracheal incision is made that is offset 45° from the orientation of the skin incision. The skin flaps and trachea flaps are interdigitated and sutured together. Next, an appropriately sized tracheostomy tube is placed. Notably, no retention sutures are used.

COMPLICATIONS AND MANAGEMENT

Tracheostomy complications can be conceptualized into groups of intraoperative, short-term, and long-term complications. Neonatal tracheostomies have high morbidity and overall mortality. Overall all-cause mortality of infants and children with tracheostomies is 1.5% to 8.9%.[26–29] One study reported tracheostomy-specific mortality at 0.7%.[26] Intraoperative complications are rare and have been reported at 3%; however, they can include accidental decannulation and loss of airway, bleeding, or vessel injury from a high-riding innominate artery, cricoid injury, skin injury, tracheal injury, or pneumothorax.[26–31] Morbidity and complications both short-term and long-term are high, reported at 19.9% to 63%.[26–29] Cardiac risk factors were independently predictive of morbidity and complications.[29]

Short-term complications include bleeding from the tracheostomy wound or thyroid gland, skin pressure necrosis, accidental decannulation with or without false tracking, tracheostomy tube mucous plugging, infection, or tracheal ulceration. A recent National Surgical Quality Improvement Program Pediatric analysis demonstrated a 7.8% rate of pneumonia and 5.8% rate of sepsis.[29] Concern for early accidental decannulation before stoma maturation often requires vigilance in tracheostomy management. Depending on the infant's risk, sedation or (in some cases) paralysis may be needed. During this time, there can be unintended pressure ulceration of the neck, chest, or chin skin from the ventilator tubing, tracheostomy tube, or tracheostomy ties.[32] Additionally, during this time, accidental decannulation via aggressive or unintentional manipulation of the trachea can occur. The tracheal retention sutures can be critical to assist with tracheostomy tube replacement or oral intubation in an emergency. Meticulous perioperative care from the surgical, nursing, and respiratory therapy team is needed to prevent morbidity.

Long-term complications can be multifactorial. An improperly sized tube or malpositioned patient can lead to tracheal granulation tissue, ulceration, erosion. Severe erosion anteriorly can cause a tracheoinnominate fistula with life-threatening bleeding. Erosion posteriorly can cause a tracheoesophageal fistula. Long-term routine tracheostomy care and follow-up are needed to help prevent these complications.[21,22,33] As the infant grows, the tracheostomy tube may become too short, thus leading to accidental decannulations that are more frequent. Tracheostomy tubes are prone to biofilm and bacterial colonization and tracheitis. Chronic infection of the tracheal cartilage can be a risk factor for secondary tracheal stenosis.

POSTOPERATIVE CARE

There are no universally agreed on standards of care for early postoperative tracheostomy care; however, there are common trends in management and care:

- Safe transport and accompaniment by the surgical team to the neonatal ICU or pediatric ICU
- Effective sign-out to the ICU team, including communicating tracheostomy type and size, cuff inflation, suction depth, and backup tracheostomy tube size; this may also include a difficult airway algorithm card placed at the bedside in case of accidental decannulation
- Frequent saline trachea suctioning to appropriate depth to prevent trachea plugging from secretions and blood
- Maintain supported ventilator tubing to prevent excessive pulling or decannulation of the tracheostomy tube

- Daily wound and skin checks for pressure ulcers, infections, and appropriate healing
- Limit patient movement and tracheostomy manipulation as much as possible during the healing process to avoid accidental decannulation
- Consider doing the first tracheostomy tube change between postoperative day 3 to 7, or as appropriate to the patient's condition
- If the first tracheostomy tube change demonstrates easy exchange with a well-healed stoma, then remove the retraction sutures and resume standard ICU tracheostomy care
- Early coordinated teaching and training of tracheostomy care to all care providers, including family and relatives.[21,22]

OUTCOMES

Besides long-term morbidity and mortality risk as previously described, there are long-term developmental outcomes to consider. Ultimate decannulation rates vary widely based on the primary indication for the tracheostomy tube. Long-term swallowing can be affected by tracheostomy tube placement or may be secondary to the primary cause that required a tracheostomy. A recent study at a single institution demonstrated 43% of infants with a tracheostomy tube were discharged with a full oral diet. The remaining 57% required some form of nasogastric, orogastric, or gastrostomy tube feeding.[34]

A large multicenter study evaluating developmental outcomes in preterm infants with tracheostomy found significant association of developmental impairment with infants receiving a tracheostomy. Neurodevelopment impairment was present in 81% of preterm infants receiving a tracheostomy with an odds ratio of 4.0. Cognitive delay was present in 77%. Motor delay was present in 68%. Neurologic impairment was present in 45%. Visual impairment was present in 4% and hearing impairment in 8%.[35]

Speech and language is believed to be impaired; however, the severity of impairment depends on initial indication for tracheostomy placement and length of tracheostomy tube presence.[36,37] Neonatal tracheostomy tubes can impede airflow through the glottis due the relative size of the tube to the airway diameter. If the airflow is restricted or there is not enough pulmonary breath support, phonation sounds will be limited in early development, which can contribute to speech and language delay. A tracheostomy speaking valve, the Passy Muir Valve, may be used to improve glottis airflow. There are some data to support the use of the Passy Muir Valve (Irvine, CA) in infants, although appropriate patient selection and close monitoring during use is needed.[38] Not all infants will be able to tolerate speaking valve use; however, awareness of the speech needs of infants and children with tracheostomy tubes is important to mitigate the impact on communication, language, and quality of life.

An additional area of neonatal tracheostomy impact is health care cost, utilization, and caregiver burden. In a study examining the total cost of tracheostomy care and related comorbidities in children over a 2-year period, the total cost was more than $60,000.[28] Because neonates are at higher risk for complications, these costs are likely higher.

SUMMARY

As there continues to be advances in neonatal care, many infants with complex chronic cardiopulmonary or neurologic conditions are having longer term survival. The indications for tracheostomy have been adapting over the years to adjust to these shifting trends.[8,9,12,15] Techniques and tracheostomy tubes have changed little.

Neonatal tracheostomy is accompanied by high risks and morbidity. A multidisciplinary approach, including the family, is needed to help monitor and mitigate the risks in these infants with complex needs. Neonatal and pediatric tracheostomies have been identified as high-morbidity procedures that need outcome improvement.[29,31] As outcomes research and data tracking are improved, there are opportunities for improved patient care, decreased morbidity and mortality, and greater standardization of care.

Best Practices

What is the current practice?

Neonatal tracheostomy

- Cardiopulmonary and neurologic disorders are the primary indications for neonatal tracheostomy.
- A vertical tracheostomy incision with retraction sutures is the predominating surgical technique.
- Neonatal tracheostomy is associated with high overall mortality and morbidity.
- Postoperative and long-term care is needed to help mitigate and manage the increased risks.
- There should be increased awareness of the neurodevelopmental impact associated with tracheostomies in all domains of development.

What changes in current practice are likely to improve outcomes?

Neonatal and pediatric tracheostomies have been identified as procedures of high morbidity with need for outcome improvement.[29,31] As outcomes research and data tracking are improved, there are opportunities for improved patient care, decreased morbidity and mortality, and greater standardization of care.

Summary statement

Tracheostomy plays a vital role in many of these conditions. Neonatal tracheostomy has significant implications and association with overall mortality, morbidity, and developmental outcomes. Although little has changed with regard to technique, there have been significant evolutions in indications, survival, complications, and technological advances. There is still a need for improved outcomes research to decrease the high associated morbidities.

REFERENCES

1. Blomstedt P. Tracheostomy in ancient Egypt. J Laryngol Otol 2014;128(8):665. Available at: http://www.ncbi.nlm.nih.gov/pubmed/25077413.
2. Donald I, Lord J. Augmented respiration. Lancet 1953;261(6755):347. Available at: https://www.sciencedirect.com/science/article/pii/S0140673653910253.
3. Mcdonald IH, Stocks JG. Prolonged nasotracheal intubation. a review of its development in a paediatric hospital. Br J Anaesth 1965;37(3):161–73. Available at: http://www.ncbi.nlm.nih.gov/pubmed/14277953.
4. Cohen S, Jones GD. Continuous positive-pressure ventilation for children with respiratory failure. Anesth Analg 1971;50(6):949–53. Available at: http://www.ncbi.nlm.nih.gov/pubmed/4942828.
5. Wailoo MP, Emery JL. Normal growth and development of the trachea. Thorax 1982;37(8):584–7. Available at: http://www.ncbi.nlm.nih.gov/pubmed/7179187.
6. Line WS, Hawkins DB, Kahlstrom EJ, et al. Tracheotomy in infants and young children: the changing perspective 1970-1985. Laryngoscope 1986;96(5):510–5. Available at: http://www.ncbi.nlm.nih.gov/pubmed/3702566.

7. Overman AE, Liu M, Kurachek SC, et al. Tracheostomy for infants requiring pro-longed mechanical ventilation: 10 years' experience. Pediatrics 2013;131(5): e1496. Available at: http://www.ncbi.nlm.nih.gov/pubmed/23569088.

8. Isaiah A, Moyer K, Pereira KD. Current trends in neonatal tracheostomy. JAMA Otolaryngol Head Neck Surg 2016;142(8):738–42.

9. Pereira KD, MacGregor AR, McDuffie CM, et al. Tracheostomy in preterm infants: current trends. Arch Otolaryngol Head Neck Surg 2003;129(12):1268–71.

10. Viswanathan S, Mathew A, Worth A, et al. Risk factors associated with the need for a tracheostomy in extremely low birth weight infants. Pediatr Pulmonol 2013; 48(2):146–50. Available at: http://onlinelibrary.wiley.com/doi/10.1002/ppul.22599/abstract.

11. Levit OL, Shabanova V, Bazzy-Asaad A, et al. Risk factors for tracheostomy requirement in extremely low birth weight infants. J Matern Fetal Neonatal Med 2017;1–6. https://doi.org/10.1080/14767058.2017.1287895.

12. McPherson ML, Shekerdemian L, Goldsworthy M, et al. A decade of pediatric tra-cheostomies: indications, outcomes, and long-term prognosis. Pediatr Pulmonol 2017;52(7):946–53. Available at: http://onlinelibrary.wiley.com/doi/10.1002/ppul.23657/abstract.

13. Murthy K, Savani RC, Lagatta JM, et al. Predicting death or tracheostomy place-ment in infants with severe bronchopulmonary dysplasia. J Perinatol 2014;34(7): 543–8. Available at: http://www.ncbi.nlm.nih.gov/pubmed/24651732.

14. Lee JH, Smith PB, Quek MBH, et al. Risk factors and in-hospital outcomes following tracheostomy in infants. J Pediatr 2016;173:44.e1. Available at: https://www.sciencedirect.com/science/article/pii/S0022347616001827.

15. Carron JD, Derkay CS, Strope GL, et al. Pediatric tracheotomies: changing indi-cations and outcomes. Laryngoscope 2000;110(7):1099–104. Available at: http://onlinelibrary.wiley.com/doi/10.1097/00005537-200007000-00006/abstract.

16. Schroeder JW, Schneider JS, Walner DL. The influence of peak airway pressure and oxygen requirement in infant tracheostomy. Int J Pediatr Otorhinolaryngol 2012;76(6):869. Available at: https://www.sciencedirect.com/science/article/pii/S0165587612001553.

17. Trachsel D, Hammer J. Indications for tracheostomy in children. Paediatr Respir Rev 2006;7(3):162–8. Available at: https://www.sciencedirect.com/science/article/pii/S1526054206004325.

18. Isayama T, Iwami H, McDonald S, et al. Association of noninvasive ventilation strategies with mortality and bronchopulmonary dysplasia among preterm in-fants: a systematic review and meta-analysis. JAMA 2016;316(6):611–24.

19. Schmölzer GM, Kumar M, Pichler G, et al. Non-invasive versus invasive respira-tory support in preterm infants at birth: systematic review and meta-analysis. BMJ 2013;347(oct17 3):f5980.

20. Subramaniam P, Ho JJ, Davis PG. Prophylactic nasal continuous positive airway pressure for preventing morbidity and mortality in very preterm infants. Cochrane Database Syst Rev 2016;(6). CD001243. Available at: http://www.ncbi.nlm.nih.gov/pubmed/27315509.

21. Boykova M. Transition from hospital to home in preterm infants and their families. J Perinat Neonatal Nurs 2016;30(3):270–2. Available at: http://ovidsp.ovid.com/ovidweb.cgi?T=JS&NEWS=n&CSC=Y&PAGE=fulltext&D=ovft&AN=00005237-201607000-00025.

22. Joseph RA. Tracheostomy in infants: parent education for home care. Neonatal Netw 2011;30(4):231–42. Available at: http://www.ncbi.nlm.nih.gov/pubmed/21729854.

23. Colman KL, Mandell DL, Simons JP. Impact of stoma maturation on pediatric tracheostomy-related complications. Arch Otolaryngol Head Neck Surg 2010; 136(5):471–4.
24. Eliashar R, Gross M, Attal P, et al. "Starplasty" prevents tracheotomy complications in infants. Int J Pediatr Otorhinolaryngol 2004;68(3):325–9. Available at: http://www.ncbi.nlm.nih.gov/pubmed/15129943.
25. Solares CA, Krakovitz P, Hirose K, et al. Starplasty: revisiting a pediatric tracheostomy technique. Otolaryngol Head Neck Surg 2004;131(5):717–22. Available at: https://www.sciencedirect.com/science/article/pii/S0194599804005285.
26. Carr MM, Poje CP, Kingston L, et al. Complications in pediatric tracheostomies. Laryngoscope 2001;111(11):1925–8. Available at: http://onlinelibrary.wiley.com/doi/10.1097/00005537-200111000-00010/abstract.
27. D'Souza JN, Levi JR, Park D, et al. Complications following pediatric tracheotomy. JAMA Otolaryngol Head Neck Surg 2016;142(5):484–8.
28. Watters K, O'Neill M, Zhu H, et al. Two-year mortality, complications, and healthcare use in children with Medicaid following tracheostomy. Laryngoscope 2016;126(11):2611–7. Available at: http://onlinelibrary.wiley.com/doi/10.1002/lary.25972/abstract.
29. Mahida JB, Asti L, Boss EF, et al. Tracheostomy placement in children younger than 2 years: 30-day outcomes using the National Surgical Quality Improvement Program Pediatric. JAMA Otolaryngol Head Neck Surg 2016;142(3):241–6.
30. Ha JF, Ostwani W, Green G. Successful conservative management of a rare complication of tracheostomy; extensive posterior tracheal false pouch. Int J Pediatr Otorhinolaryngol 2016;90:54–7.
31. Shah RK, Stey AM, Jatana KR, et al. Identification of opportunities for quality improvement and outcome measurement in pediatric otolaryngology. JAMA Otolaryngol Head Neck Surg 2014;140(11):1019–26.
32. Hart CK, Tawfik KO, Meinzen-Derr J, et al. A randomized controlled trial of velcro versus standard twill ties following pediatric tracheotomy. Laryngoscope 2017; 127(9):1996–2001. Available at: http://onlinelibrary.wiley.com/doi/10.1002/lary.26608/abstract.
33. Gergin O, Adil E, Kawai K, et al. Routine airway surveillance in pediatric tracheostomy patients. Int J Pediatr Otorhinolaryngol 2017;97:1–4. Available at: https://www.sciencedirect.com/science/article/pii/S0165587617301118.
34. Joseph RA, Evitts P, Bayley EW, et al. Oral feeding outcome in infants with a tracheostomy. J Pediatr Nurs 2016. https://doi.org/10.1016/j.pedn.2016.12.012.
35. DeMauro SB, D'Agostino JA, Bann C, et al. Developmental outcomes of very preterm infants with tracheostomies. J Pediatr 2014;164(6):1310.e2. Available at: http://www.ncbi.nlm.nih.gov/pubmed/24472229.
36. Hill BP, Singer LT. Speech and language development after infant tracheostomy. J Speech Hear Disord 1990;55(1):15–20. Available at: http://jshd.asha.org/cgi/content/abstract/55/1/15.
37. Jiang D, Morrison GAJ. The influence of long-term tracheostomy on speech and language development in children. Int J Pediatr Otorhinolaryngol 2003;67:S220. Available at: https://www.sciencedirect.com/science/article/pii/S0165587603002921.
38. Engleman SG, Turnage-Carrier C. Tolerance of the Passy-Muir speaking valve in infants and children less than 2 years of age. Pediatr Nurs 1997;23(6):571. Available at: http://www.ncbi.nlm.nih.gov/pubmed/9429513.

Neonatal Stridor
Diagnosis and Management

Jay Bhatt, MD[a], Jeremy D. Prager, MD, MBA[b],*

KEYWORDS

- Neonatal respiratory distress • Neonatal stridor • Laryngeal obstruction
- Tracheal anomalies

KEY POINTS

- Stridor is defined by a high-pitched respiratory sound that signals an airway anomaly.
- Stridor is a result of obstruction at the laryngeal and/or at the tracheobronchial levels.
- The evaluation and management of neonates with stridor is the focus of the this article

INTRODUCTION

Respiratory distress is a common problem in neonates, estimated to be present in 7% of all newborns.[1] Unfortunately, more than 46% of all child deaths are among newborn infants, three-quarters of which occur in the first week of life. Stridor is among most common presenting signs of respiratory distress in newborns. Therefore, early recognition of stridor and a thorough workup are paramount in avoiding an adverse outcome.

Stridor is defined by a high-pitched respiratory sound that can be present on inspiration, expiration, or both, that signals an airway anomaly. Stridor may be an individual sign or can present with 1 or more signs of increased work of breathing, such as tachypnea, nasal flaring, chest retractions, or grunting.[2–4] Often, these are compensatory mechanisms for hypercarbia, hypoxemia, or acidosis (both metabolic and respiratory) secondary to the process that may be creating the neonate's stridor. These constellations of signs are common but nonspecific findings in a large variety of respiratory, cardiovascular, metabolic, or systemic diseases,[2,3,5] which should prompt further workup when accompanied with stridor.

The cause of stridor and respiratory distress in newborns is wide-ranging and includes many systemic causes.[4] These include intrathoracic causes, both medical

Disclosure Statement: None.
[a] Department of Pediatric Otolaryngology, Children's Hospital Colorado, 13123 E 16th Avenue, B-455, Aurora, CO 80045, USA; [b] Department of Otolaryngology, University of Colorado School of Medicine, 12631 E. 17th Avenue, B-205, Aurora, CO 80045, USA
* Corresponding author.
E-mail address: jeremy.prager@childrenscolorado.org

Clin Perinatol 45 (2018) 817–831
https://doi.org/10.1016/j.clp.2018.07.015   **perinatology.theclinics.com**

and surgical; extrathoracic pathologic conditions in the central nervous system, skeletal system, and/or the gastrointestinal system; systemic causes, such as sepsis or electrolyte imbalance; and acquired or congenital causes in the airway.

Pathologic conditions in the upper airway begin at the nasal level, with conditions such as neonatal rhinitis, piriform aperture stenosis, and choanal atresia. At the oropharyngeal level, obstruction can result from anomalies such as micrognathia or macroglossia. Pathologic conditions at the previously mentioned anatomic levels do not cause stridor and thus are not further discussed. Stridor is typically a result of obstruction at the laryngeal and/or at the tracheobronchial levels, a discussion of which is the focus of this article.

EVALUATION

Evaluation of a newborn with stridor, as of any patient, begins with obtaining a thorough yet relevant history. The history can be obtained in the usual fashion as long as the neonate is clinically stable and does not need urgent intervention.

History should include the quality, the time of onset, and contributing and relieving factors of the stridor. Of particular importance are the baby's antenatal, perinatal, and birth history; history of prior procedures and surgeries; and history of intubation. If the neonate has been intubated, knowing the size, cuff status, and length of intubation is valuable. Additional data about supplemental oxygen and its delivery methods should be obtained.

If hospitalized, further relevant information can be gathered from nursing staff and respiratory therapists in regard to the neonate's stridor and respiratory distress, including positional changes, feeding issues, and the exact nature of distress associated with each episode. Use of technology can be helpful because many parents in the twenty-first century video record such events in their children. Thus, it is important ask parents if they have such recordings and review them during the evaluation.

After obtaining general information, relevant otolaryngologic history should become the focus of the history taking. These includes signs and symptoms such as

- Nasal congestion
- Rhinorrhea
- Dyspnea
- Cyanotic episodes
- Feeding difficulties, such as gagging, choking, coughing, vomiting, or refluxing with feeds
- Failure to thrive or gain adequate weight
- Difficulty sleeping.

Thereafter, a detailed physical examination should be performed. It should include external impression for gross deformities in the head and neck, and chest. Additionally, a thorough evaluation should be performed for

- Other external deformities
- Breathing sounds (**Table 1**)
  - Work of breathing, with additional signs of
    - Nasal flaring
    - Chest retractions
    - Perioral cyanosis
    - Suprasternal and subcostal retractions
    - Abdominal muscle usage
- Presence of mucous or excessive secretions
- Anterior nasal stenosis, mucous, or masses (visualized with anterior rhinoscopy).

Table 1
Breathing sounds: description of common breathing sounds and their usual causes

Sound	Quality	Causes
Stertor	Snoring sound, mid-pitched	• Nasopharyngeal obstruction (eg, choanal atresia) • Redundant upper airway tissue • Oropharyngeal lesions
Stridor	High-pitched	• Inspiratory: supraglottic (eg, laryngomalacia) • Biphasic: glottic or subglottic (eg, congenital glottis web) • Expiratory: distal tracheal airway (eg, tracheomalacia)
Wheezing	High-pitched, whistling; typically expiratory	• Lower airway obstruction (eg, reactive airway disease)
Grunting	Low-pitched or mid-pitched, sudden closure of glottis during expiration	• Compensatory for poor pulmonary compliance due to transient tachypnea of newborn, pneumonia, atelectasis

Finally, a flexible suction catheter should be passed through each nasal passage, typically 5-6 French, to ensure an easy passage and patent choanae. Care should be taken with children with craniofacial abnormalities and nasal masses because of the high risk of skull base defects.

WORKUP AND MANAGEMENT

Management of a newborn with stridor, with or without respiratory distress, begins with establishing a safe airway and stabilizing the baby, if indicated. Noninvasive or invasive airway interventions can be used, as needed. Of note, oxygen delivery with helium in the form of heliox (nitrogen 80%, oxygen 20%) can also be used in certain situations to deliver high flows of oxygen through narrow and partially obstructed airway passages by improving laminar air flow.

Laboratory analysis typically has low yield in the workup of neonatal stridor, unless an infectious cause is suspected. Similarly, the role of imaging is limited in the acute setting but may be helpful for further diagnostic workup and before decision-making. Imaging is indicated in select cases, particularly in evaluation of congenital anomalies. Computed tomography (CT) and MRI can be used to further delineate the anatomy around laryngoceles or congenital saccular cysts (see later discussion). Prenatal ultrasound and MRI are valuable in the diagnosis of congenital high airway obstruction syndrome (CHAOS). Contrast imaging and echocardiography are also useful in the diagnosis and management of vascular causes of tracheomalacia. These can be ordered based on preendoscopic index of suspicion or on endoscopic findings but are generally not the first steps in diagnostic workup. However, no single imaging modality is the be-all and end-all of neonatal stridor, and diagnostic imaging must be catered to the suspected pathologic conditions. The role of certain imaging modalities in specific cases is discussed when indicated.

Flexible fiberoptic laryngoscopy has become the workhorse of evaluation of stridor. It can help assess the dynamic movement of the laryngeal structures in a quick and reliable fashion, typically without the need for sedation or anesthesia. A direct laryngoscope with bronchoscopy may also be indicated in certain patients in whom glottic or subglottic pathologic conditions are suspected. In these cases, a detailed plan should be made in advance with the anesthesia team to protect and share the airway to maximize the chances of favorable outcomes.

Causes of Neonatal Stridor

Neonatal stridor can be broadly differentiated by its characteristic sounds: inspiratory, expiratory, or biphasic. Inspiratory stridor suggests supraglottic pathologic conditions, biphasic stridor is heard in glottic or subglottic pathologic conditions, and expiratory stridor is more common in tracheal pathologic conditions. These characteristics are broad and certainly should not be used to exclude pathologic conditions. Rather, they serve to narrow the focus of a clinician's evaluation. Additionally, given that the structure of the larynx can be divided in 3 areas (supraglottic, glottic, and subglottic), categorization of neonatal stridor can follow this anatomic division.

The following sections explore common pathologic conditions seen in each anatomic location of the larynx.

Supraglottic Causes of Stridor

The presence of inspiratory stridor indicates supraglottic pathologic conditions. Potential supraglottic pathologic conditions in neonates are

- Laryngomalacia
- Congenital laryngeal saccular cyst
- CHAOS.

Laryngomalacia

Laryngomalacia is considered to be the most common congenital laryngeal anomaly and the most common cause of neonatal stridor, accounting for up to 70% of cases.[6] Most often, neonates present in the first few weeks of life, and symptoms often resolve by 18 months of age without intervention. Infants with laryngomalacia have a characteristic high-pitched inspiratory stridor, which is worsened with supine positioning and feeding. There are several theories about the pathophysiology of laryngomalacia: neurologic, anatomic, and cartilaginous.

The neurologic theory suggests that the stridor is secondary to neuromuscular discoordination resulting from sensory dysfunction.[7] The obstruction and the resulting stridor are thus thought to be secondary to the collapse of supraglottic tissue caused by this abnormal laryngeal tone. The anatomic theory suggests that differences in patient's anatomy create supraglottic collapse.[8] At baseline, an infant's larynx is in a higher position at birth to facilitate spontaneous breathing, prevent aspiration, and to allow for simultaneous feeding and breathing.[9] However, the position and the length of an infant's epiglottis, and the addition of a short aryepiglottic fold may play a role in the supraglottic collapse during inspiration.[8] In addition, the cartilaginous theory suggests that the pliability of the infant cartilage may worsen these 2 pathogeneses, leading to the collapse that yields the stridor and airway obstruction.

The contribution of gastroesophageal reflux has been intensely studied and shown to contribute to symptoms of laryngomalacia. Gastroesophageal reflux is the most common comorbidity found in patients with laryngomalacia.[10–12] As a result, medical management to control stomach acid in these infants is of paramount importance according to some studies. However, use of proton-pump inhibitors to control gastric acid secretion remains controversial[14] both for their use in laryngomalacia and the increasing evidence for potential harm.[15]

Flexible fiberoptic laryngoscopy is the modality of choice in the evaluation of infants suspected to have stridor secondary to laryngomalacia. It is thought to have nearly 90% accuracy in diagnosis, regardless of the operator.[16] The flexible laryngoscopy reveals certain findings that are characteristic of laryngomalacia. These include

- Prolapse of redundant arytenoid mucosa
- Short aryepiglottic folds
- Omega-shaped epiglottis
- Posteriorly displaced epiglottis.

Laryngomalacia usually resolves by 18 months of age; therefore, most patients do not require surgical intervention.[13] Stridor; difficulty feeding; obstructive breathing by history, examination, or polysomnography; and failure to thrive are the most common indications for a supraglottoplasty.[10,17] Other surgical indications include brief resolved unexplained events (formerly apparent life-threatening events) and desaturations. When surgical intervention is required, cold steel, microdebrider, laser, and the coblator are the most often used tools. Supraglottoplasty is a safe and successful procedure[13,18] but can lead to transient worsened swallowing dysfunction.[19] The most commonly identified source of surgical failure is severe reflux symptoms. Technique, age, and gender have no bearing on outcomes.[17,20,21] Additionally, patients with multiple comorbidities, such as associated syndromes and neurologic conditions, are more likely to fail[18] and may need further interventions, including revisions surgery or a tracheostomy.[13,21]

Congenital laryngeal saccular cyst

A congenital laryngeal saccular cyst is an abnormal dilation of the saccule that can cause airway obstruction and stridor. It is a relatively rare entity but should be recognized because it can lead to supraglottic prolapse, similar to the prolapse seen in laryngomalacia.[22,23] The rarity, the potential for severe presentation, and anatomic location make saccular cysts lethal causes of respiratory distress. Most commonly, neonates present with stridor, respiratory distress, failure to thrive, poor feeding, and cyanotic spells. The typical age of presentation is 16 days to 8 months.[22] Coexistent laryngomalacia is a common finding.

MRI and CT imaging or an ultrasound can be obtained for diagnostic purposes. However, motion artifact of the larynx can make MRI imaging without heavy sedation difficult. Flexible fiberoptic laryngoscopy is a very useful tool in the diagnosis of these lesions and can be used with direct laryngoscopy.[24]

Most patients achieve complete remission following surgical intervention with as marsupialization, aspiration, or extirpation. Aspiration carries the highest risk of recurrence,[25] and extirpation may require an external approach. Therefore, marsupialization, which carries a very low rate of recurrence, is often the surgical treatment of choice.[24,26]

Congenital high airway obstruction syndrome

CHAOS is defined as obstruction diagnosed in utero by ultrasound with characteristic findings.[27] A combination of polyhydramnios, tracheal dilation, enlarged and echogenic lungs, and flattening or inversion of the diaphragm can be seen on fetal ultrasound or MRI.[28–30]

The most common cause of CHAOS is laryngeal atresia.[31] Even with a timely diagnosis, only a small number of newborns survive the condition. In suspected CHAOS patients, ex utero intrapartum treatment (EXIT) is used in delivery. Newborns typically require a surgical airway within 1 hour of birth because they cannot be intubated tracheally. CHAOS patients can be divided in 3 clinical presentations. The mildest presentation is near-complete high upper obstruction, followed by complete atresia with the presence of a tracheoesophageal fistula. The most severe presentation is a complete laryngeal atresia without an esophageal fistula.[32] The management of the airway, beyond tracheostomy on EXIT, is complex, challenging, and continues to evolve.

Glottic Causes of Stridor

Glottic pathologic conditions most commonly cause biphasic stridor, even though occasional isolated inspiratory or expiratory stridor may occur. Glottic pathologic conditions include

- Vocal fold paralysis (VFP), unilateral or bilateral
- Laryngeal web
- Laryngeal atresia
- Laryngeal cleft.

Laryngeal webs

Developmental abnormalities such as atresia and webs are generally recognized in the first few days of life. A normal larynx is formed by the dissolution and autolysis of epithelial tissue from the dorsal to the ventral part of the larynx, which is affected in these conditions. The infants present with dyspnea and dysphonia, although some have aphonia, as well as stridor and respiratory distress.

Laryngeal web is a spectrum of laryngeal atresia, which is classified in 3 main categories[33,34] ranging from complete atresia to congenital glottic web. The most severe form, type 1, is the complete atresia of the larynx with a small duct along dorsal border, which is a seventh-week developmental deformity. Type 2, which tends to be less severe, is a supraglottic obstruction separating the vestibule and the infraglottic cavity, occurring during eighth week of fetal development. Insults in the ninth week of development cause a type 3 laryngeal atresia, which is the most common. This anomaly is a perforated membrane of variable thickness at the level of the vocal folds and is commonly known as congenital web or glottic web.[33]

In 1954, Holinger and colleagues[35] first described type 3 laryngeal atresia and coined the term congenital glottic web. In 1985, Cohen[36] developed a classification system for glottic webs, describing them in 4 different categories based on the degree of obstruction. Type 1 is the least severe, with less than 35% obstruction, and type 4 is the worst, with up to 99% obstruction. Type 2 has 35% to 50% involvement, whereas type 3 has 50% to 75% (**Fig. 1**).[36]

The management of patients with glottic webs is based on the degree of obstruction and associated anomalies. Type 1 and 2 webs are operated on only in cases of symptomatic airway obstruction.[36] Types 3 and 4 are more challenging to manage and often require an early tracheostomy. Typically, an open approach to the airway is required to manage these definitively.[33]

Vocal fold paralysis

VFP is the second most common abnormality in the pediatric larynx, after laryngomalacia. Neonates with cord paralysis present with weak cough, weak cry, dysphonia, aphonia, dysphagia, aspiration, and even airway compromise. If unilateral paralysis is present, the most common presenting sign is dysphonia.[37] Airway compromise tends to be more common in those with bilateral VFP. These infants are typically more likely to present with cyanosis and apnea.[37]

The most common causes of VFP in the pediatric population are cardiac surgery (68.8%), idiopathic (21.0%), and neurologic (7.4%).[38] In bilateral cases, they are idiopathic causes (30%), prolonged intubation (25%), and neurologic causes (22%).[39] In

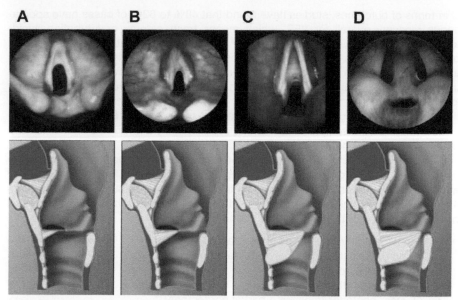

Fig. 1. Cohen's classification of congenital glottic web. (*A*) Type 1 glottic web, less than 35%. (*B*) Type 2 glottic web, 35% to 50%. (*C*) Type 3 glottic web, 50% to 75% with subglottic stenosis due to involvement of anterior cricoid. (*D*) Type 4 glottic web, up to 99% with subglottic stenosis due to involvement of anterior cricoid. (*From* de Trey LA, Lambercy K, Monnier P, et al. Management of severe congenital laryngeal webs - a 12 year review. Int J Pediatr Otorhinolaryngol 2016;86:83; with permission.)

cases of prolonged intubation, tube position, particularly excessively large tubes, contributes to cord weakness. In most patients with neurologic causes of VFP, the protrusion of the brainstem through the foramen magnum into the spinal canal, such as that caused by an Arnold-Chiari malformation, is thought to stretch and compress the vagus nerve.[40] Birth trauma can also contribute to VFP because the use of delivery forceps can compress or stretch both recurrent laryngeal nerves.[41] In cases of unilateral VFP, the left side is most commonly affected (66.8%), followed by bilateral (25.3%) and the right side (7.9%).[38] Across all studies, cardiac surgery is consistently among most common factors contributing to unilateral VFP, resulting in a 1.7% to 67% rate of paralysis.[42] This wide range of paralysis results from the type and extent of surgery because surgery around the aortic arch possesses the highest risk, whereas other areas have lower risk.[42] However, importantly, subglottic stenosis is the most common sequelae of cardiac surgery, rather than VFP.[43]

The presence of a safe airway and feeding are the most pressing concerns in infants with VFP. Most patients with unilateral VFP may need no to very little supplemental oxygen or ventilator support. However, in 1 study, the investigators found that greater than half of subjects required a tracheostomy, particularly in the case of bilateral VFP.[44] Notably, most of those in cohorts that need a tracheostomy had other comorbidities or coexisting upper airway disease.[44,45]

Many neonates and infants with VFP have issues with feeding. There are generally no long-term effects from vocal fold immobility with regard to pneumonia.[46] However, there is increased risk of readmission for feeding difficulty or poor weight gain. Consequently, some investigators estimate that, because of feeding issues, up to 52% of unilateral and bilateral VFP patients may require a gastrostomy tube for long-term management.[38]

In terms of outcomes, studies have found that 48% to 62% of cases have spontaneous recovery overall for VFP, which means tracheostomy or intubation avoidance.[39,45] Comparatively, iatrogenic VFP has the lowest rate of recovery.[45] In particular, ligation of a patent ductus arteriosus results in paralysis up to 67% of cases and has a low 3% recovery at 3.6 years mean follow-up.[47] The investigators think that this procedure likely causes complete disruption of the nerve, resulting in extremely low rates of recovery. However, in general, up to an 82% recovery rate is seen in patients with cardiac surgery, which can take a median of 6 months or more.[43,48,49] However, in those patients who fail to recover, even after 3 years, 47% continue to have dysphagia and 20% have dysphonia.

Surgical management to address the glottic obstruction can be undertaken, particularly if the problem persists. The success of decannulation after tracheostomy or avoidance of tracheostomy is variable in these patients after surgery, ranging from 40% to 100%.[50] Although the details and merits of each of these is debated and beyond the scope of this article, they are as follows:

- Arytenoidectomy with suture lateralization
- Carbon dioxide (CO_2) laser arytenoidectomy[51]
- Posterior cordotomy[52]
- Combination of the previous 2[53]
- CO_2 laser posterior transverse partial cordectomy[54]
- Suture lateralization[55]
- Laryngeal reinnervation
- Endoscopic anterior and posterior cricoid split.[56]

Laryngeal cleft

A laryngeal cleft is an anomalous connection between the larynx and the hypopharynx thought to be secondary to sixth branchial arch issues. Patients with laryngeal clefts present with stridor; chronic cough; aspiration; and, often, recurrent respiratory infections.

The condition was first classified by Benjamin and Inglis.[57] This system is currently the most commonly used (**Fig. 2**):

- Type 1: Secondary to incomplete formation of interarytenoid muscle, with or without normal interarytenoid mucosa
- Type 2: Incomplete formation of posterior corticoid cartilage
- Type 3: Incomplete formation of the tracheoesophageal septum distal to cricoid
- Type 4: The extension of type 3 into the thorax.

Even though a laryngeal cleft can occur in isolation, there are several syndromes associated with the condition. The most common syndromes include

- Opitz-Frias
- Vertebral, Anal, Tracheo-Esophageal and Renal anomalies (VATER) and Vertebral defects, anal atresia, cardiac defects, tracheo-esophageal fistula, renal anomalies, and limb abnormalities (VACTERL)
- Pallister Hall
- CHARGE (coloboma, heart defects, atresia choanae [also known as choanal atresia], growth retardation, genital abnormalities, and ear abnormalities).

The diagnosis of a laryngeal cleft can be definitely confirmed via a direct laryngoscopy. During the endoscopy, the interarytenoid area is palpated with a blunt laryngeal probe to evaluate the depth and presence of laryngeal cleft. Swallow imaging is a useful adjunct. A modified barium swallow (MBS) is particularly useful because most

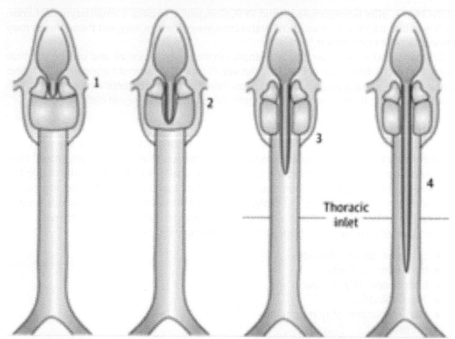

Fig. 2. The 4 types of laryngeal clefts. (1) Secondary to incomplete formation of interarytenoid muscle, with or without normal interarytenoid mucosa. (2) Incomplete formation of posterior corticoid cartilage. (3) Incomplete formation of the tracheoesophageal septum distal to cricoid. (4) The extension of type 3 into the thorax. (*From* Benjamin B, Inglis A. Minor congenital laryngeal clefts: diagnosis and classification. Ann Otol Rhinol Laryngol 1989;98(6):417–20.)

patients with type 1 and type 2 laryngeal clefts will have aspiration on MBS.[58] A functional endoscopic evaluation of swallowing can be an adjunct because it provides a dynamic view of aspiration[59] and can help guide swallow therapy. However, in patients who are intermittent aspirators, both of these diagnostics studies may show normal swallowing and may yield little diagnostic value.

The goals of management in patients with laryngeal cleft include reducing aspiration, improving nutrition, and decreasing pulmonary sequelae of the disease. Patients with type 1 laryngeal clefts can be managed conservatively, with dietary modifications and reducing GERD. For the higher grade clefts or type 1 clefts that fail medical management, surgical therapy for aspiration is a viable option.[60,61]

Subglottic Causes of Stridor

Subglottic pathologic conditions typically yield a biphasic stridor. Common causes of subglottic pathologic conditions are

- Subglottic stenosis
- Subglottic hemangioma.

Subglottic stenosis

Subglottic stenosis is worth mentioning in the setting of neonatal respiratory distress. As previously discussed, subglottic stenosis can be categorized as congenital or acquired. Congenital subglottic stenosis is the third most common congenital anomaly of the larynx, after laryngomalacia and VFP. Congenital implies a small laryngeal lumen with no other apparent cause; however, some investigators suggest these cases may have a familial component.[62]

Congenital subglottic stenosis is typically cartilaginous in nature and can be elliptical (most common), flattened, or clefted.[63] An elliptical cricoid is most frequently seen[63] and occurs when the transverse diameter is less than the anteroposterior diameter (**Fig. 3**).[63] Not infrequently, these may be associated with posterior laryngeal cleft.[64]

Subglottic hemangioma

Subglottic hemangioma is a rare but important consideration in infants presenting with stridor. Infants with subglottic hemangioma can have up to a 50% morality rate,[65] thus it should be suspected in this group of patients. Typically, an infant presents during the proliferative phase with symptomatic biphasic stridor and can have a barking cough as commonly seen in croup. Notably, they also follow the same pattern of growth as infantile hemangioma patients and may be managed as so in many cases.

Management options for subglottic hemangioma includes[66]

- Systemic corticosteroids
- Intralesion steroids
- Endoscopic CO_2 excision
- Tracheostomy
- Open resection of hemangioma
- Propranolol.

Because subglottic hemangioma often follows the same pattern of growth as infantile hemangioma, propranolol use has become popular as the primary management tool in recent years. Multiple large studies have demonstrated that it can be used as first-line therapy in most cases[67–69] or as an adjunct with steroids or tracheostomy.[70] However, some clinicians have reported inconsistent results when used as first line-treatment,[71] which can be decreased with increasing doses of propranolol, up to 3 mg/kg per day.[72] However, certain patients may have a failed response or subsequent regrowth, which may ultimately require laryngotracheal reconstruction.[73]

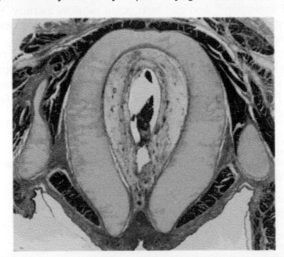

Fig. 3. A horizontal section of a cricoid ring with an elliptical lumen and a submucous cleft of the posterior cricoid lamina. (*From* Schroeder JW Jr, Holinger LD. Congenital laryngeal stenosis. Otolaryngol Clin North Am 2008;41(5):865–75.)

Tracheal Causes of Stridor

Tracheomalacia

Neonates with tracheomalacia can present with a range of respiratory symptoms, including persistent barky cough, wheezing, dyspnea, and biphasic stridor.[74] Tracheomalacia can be primary if caused by intrinsic alterations of the tracheal cartilage or the trachealis muscle. Secondary tracheomalacia occurs in the setting of extrinsic compression, such as from a vascular compression, or due to another anomaly, such as a tracheoesophageal fistula. Management options are varied and include observation or a widening range of surgical interventions.[75,76]

Tracheomalacia or compromised lumen from coaptation secondary to vascular compression commonly occurs in the

1. Double aortic arch
2. Right aortic arch
3. Anomalous innominate artery
4. Anomalous left common carotid
5. Pulmonary artery sling
6. Retroesophageal right subclavian artery.

The stridor is typically biphasic in nature, secondary to external compression of the trachea. The need for repair, similar to primary tracheomalacia, takes place in patients with severe symptoms.

Complete tracheal rings and congenital tracheal stenosis

Most patients with complete tracheal rings are symptomatic from birth and may have associated anomalies. These infant's rings typically have symptoms of biphasic stridor; respiratory distress; or, in some cases, progressive exertional dyspnea. Rarely, a child may be undiagnosed until intubation is needed for other purposes.[77] Similarly, congenital tracheal stenosis is a relatively rare condition that presents in the neonatal period with respiratory distress and stridor with cyanosis within first hours to days of life and can be associated with pulmonary agenesis. This pathologic condition varies in location of stenosis, the severity, and the length of the stenotic segments.[78] The true incidence of these conditions is not known. Most patients require a slide tracheoplasty, particularly in cases of respiratory failure or worsening status.[79]

SUMMARY

Stridor in a neonate can occur due to a range of pathologic conditions in the larynx, which should be evaluated promptly. Although the most common causes of neonatal stridor do not cause immediate harm to the neonate, there are potentially life-threatening causes that can cause rapid deterioration and airway compromise. Therefore, a thorough evaluation of the supraglottis, glottis, subglottis, and the tracheal airway are indicated for optimal outcome.

Best Practices

For perinatologists caring for neonates with stridor, stabilization of the baby's airway status and consultation with pediatric otolaryngology may be warranted. Typically, no direct imaging is indicated acutely, and diagnostic imaging must be catered to the suspected pathologic condition. Endoscopic visualization of the airway is the mainstay of diagnosis and can help guide further management.

Ultimately, prompt evaluation of stridor to evaluate for the life-threatening causes done in a targeted, multidisciplinary fashion, yields the best outcome.

REFERENCES

1. World Health Organization. "Newborns: reducing mortality". Geneva (Switzerland): World Health Organization; 2017. Accessed November 6, 2018.
2. Edwards MO, Kotecha SJ, Kotecha S. Respiratory distress of the term newborn infant. Paediatr Respir Rev 2013;14(1):29–36.
3. Warren JB, Anderson JM. Newborn respiratory disorders. Pediatr Rev 2010; 31(12):487–95 [quiz: 496].
4. Reuter S, Moser C, Baack M. Respiratory distress in the newborn. Pediatr Rev 2014;35(10):417–28 [quiz: 429].
5. West JB, editor. Respiratory physiology: the essentials. Baltimore (MD): Williams & Wilkins; 2012.
6. Daniel SJ. The upper airway: congenital malformations. Paediatr Respir Rev 2006;7:S260–3.
7. Thompson DM. Abnormal sensorimotor integrative function of the larynx in congenital laryngomalacia: a new theory of etiology. Laryngoscope 2007;117: 1–33.
8. Manning SC, Inglis AF, Mouzakes J, et al. Laryngeal anatomic differences in pediatric patients with severe laryngomalacia. Arch Otolaryngol Head Neck Surg 2005;131:340–3.
9. Lieberman DE, McCarthy RC, Hiiemae KM, et al. Ontogeny of postnatal hyoid and larynx descent in humans. Arch Oral Biol 2001;46:117–28.
10. Garritano FG, Carr MM. Characteristics of patients undergoing supraglottoplasty for laryngomalacia. Int J Pediatr Otorhinolaryngol 2014;78(7):1095–100.
11. Simons JP, Greenberg LL, Mehta DK, et al. Laryngomalacia and swallowing function in children. Laryngoscope 2016;126(2):478–84.
12. Chandra RK, Gerber ME, Holinger LD. Histological insight into the pathogenesis of severe laryngomalacia. Int J Pediatr Otorhinolaryngol 2001;61:31–8.
13. Thompson DM. Laryngomalacia: factors that influence disease severity and outcomes of management. Curr Opin Otolaryngol Head Neck Surg 2010;18(6): 564–70.
14. Apps JR, Flint JD, Wacogne I. Towards evidence based medicine for paediatricians. Question 1. Does anti-reflux therapy improve symptoms in infants with laryngomalacia? Arch Dis Child 2012;97:385–7.
15. Angelidou A, Bell K, Gupta M, et al. Implementation of a guideline to decrease use of acid-suppressing medications in the NICU. Pediatrics 2017;140(6) [pii: e20171715].
16. Lima TM, Goncalves DU, Goncalves LV, et al. Flexible nasolaryngoscopy accuracy in laryngomalacia diagnosis. Braz J Otorhinolaryngol 2008;74:29–32.
17. Ramprasad VH, Ryan MA, Farjat AE, et al. Practice patterns in supraglottoplasty and perioperative care. Int J Pediatr Otorhinolaryngol 2016;86:118–23.
18. Durvasula VS, Lawson BR, Bower CM, et al. Supraglottoplasty outcomes in neurologically affected and syndromic children. JAMA Otolaryngol Head Neck Surg 2014;140(8):704–11.
19. Chun RH, Wittkopf M, Sulman C, et al. Transient swallowing dysfunction in typically developing children following supraglottoplasty for laryngomalacia. Int J Pediatr Otorhinolaryngol 2014;78(11):1883–5.
20. Douglas CM, Shafi A, Higgins G, et al. Risk factors for failure of supraglottoplasty. Int J Pediatr Otorhinolaryngol 2014;78(9):1485–8.

21. Hwang E, Chung J, MacCormick J, et al. Success of supraglottoplasty for severe laryngomalacia: the experience from Northeastern Ontario, Canada. Int J Pediatr Otorhinolaryngol 2013;77(7):1103–6.
22. Sands NB, Anand SM, Manoukian JJ. Series of congenital vallecular cysts: a rare yet potentially fatal cause of upper airway obstruction and failure to thrive in the newborn. J Otolaryngol Head Neck Surg 2009;38(1):6–10.
23. Yao TC, Chiu CY, Wu KC, et al. Failure to thrive caused by the coexistence of vallecular cyst, laryngomalacia and gastroesophageal reflux in an infant. Int J Pediatr Otorhinolaryngol 2004;68(11):1459–64.
24. Suzuki J, Hashimoto S, Watanabe K, et al. Congenital vallecular cyst in an infant: case report and review of 52 recent cases. J Laryngol Otol 2011;125(11):1199–203.
25. Tibesar RJ, Thompson DM. Apnea spells in an infant with vallecular cyst. Ann Otol Rhinol Laryngol 2003;112:821–4.
26. Pak MW, Woo JK, van Hasselt CA. Congenital laryngeal cysts: current approach to management. J Laryngol Otol 1996;110(9):854–6.
27. Hedrick MH, Ferro MM, Filly RA, et al. Congenital high airway obstruction syndrome (CHAOS): a potential for perinatal intervention. J Pediatr Surg 1994;29(2):271–4.
28. Gupta K, Venkatesan B, Manoharan KS, et al. CHAOS: prenatal imaging findings with post mortem contrast radiographic correlation. J Radiol Case Rep 2016;10(8):39–49.
29. Roybal J, Liechty K, Hedrick H, et al. Predicting the severity of congenital high airway obstruction syndrome. J Pediatr Surg 2010;45(8):1633–9.
30. Sharma R, Dey AK, Alam S, et al. A series of congenital high airway obstruction syndrome – classic imaging findings. J Clin Diagn Res 2016;10(3):TD07–9.
31. Vidaeff AC, Szmuk P, Mastrobattista JM, et al. More or less CHAOS: case report and literature review suggesting the existence of a distinct subtype of congenital high airway obstruction syndrome. Ultrasound Obstet Gynecol 2007;30:114–7.
32. Hartnick CJ, Rutter M, Lang F, et al. Congenital high airway obstruction syndrome and airway reconstruction: an evolving paradigm. Arch Otolaryngol Head Neck Surg 2002;128(5):567–70.
33. de Trey LA, Lambercy K, Monnier P, et al. Management of severe congenital laryngeal webs - a 12 year review. Int J Pediatr Otorhinolaryngol 2016;86:82–6.
34. Zaw-Tun HI. Development of congenital laryngeal atresias and clefts. Ann Otol Rhinol Laryngol 1988;97(4 Pt 1):353–8.
35. Holinger PH, Johnson KC, Schiller F. Congenital anomalies of the larynx. Ann Otol Rhinol Laryngol 1954;63(3):581–606.
36. Cohen SR. Congenital glottic webs in children. A retrospective review of 51 patients. Ann Otol Rhinol Laryngol Suppl 1985;121:2–16.
37. Rosin DF, Handler SD, Potsic WP, et al. Vocal cord paralysis in children. Laryngoscope 1990;100:1174–9.
38. Jabbour J, Martin T, Beste D, et al. Pediatric vocal fold immobility: natural history and the need for long-term follow-up. JAMA Otolaryngol Head Neck Surg 2014;140(5):428–33.
39. Hsu J, Tibbetts KM, Wu D, et al. Swallowing function in pediatric patients with bilateral vocal fold immobility. Int J Pediatr Otorhinolaryngol 2017;93:37–41.
40. Chen EY, Inglis AF. Bilateral vocal cord paralysis in children. Otolaryngol Clin North Am 2008;41(5):889–901.
41. Hughes CA, Harley EH, Milmoe G, et al. Birth trauma in the head and neck. Arch Otolaryngol Head Neck Surg 1999;125(2):193–9.

42. Dewan K, Cephus C, Owczarzak V, et al. Incidence and implication of vocal fold paresis following neonatal cardiac surgery. Laryngoscope 2012;122(12):2781–5.

43. Khariwala SS, Lee WT, Koltai PJ. Laryngotracheal consequences of pediatric cardiac surgery. Arch Otolaryngol Head Neck Surg 2005;131(4):336–9.

44. Miyamoto RC, Parikh SR, Gellad W, et al. Bilateral congenital vocal cord paralysis: a 16-year institutional review. Otolaryngol Head Neck Surg 2005;133(2):241–5.

45. Daya H, Hosni A, Bejar-Solar I, et al. Pediatric vocal fold paralysis: a long-term retrospective study. Arch Otolaryngol Head Neck Surg 2000;126(1):21–5.

46. Richter AL, Ongkasuwan J, Ocampo EC. Long-term follow-up of vocal fold movement impairment and feeding after neonatal cardiac surgery. Int J Pediatr Otorhinolaryngol 2016;83:211–4.

47. Nichols BG, Jabbour J, Hehir DA, et al. Recovery of vocal fold immobility following isolated patent ductus arteriosus ligation. Int J Pediatr Otorhinolaryngol 2014;78(8):1316–9.

48. Truong MT, Messner AH, Kerschner JE, et al. Pediatric vocal fold paralysis after cardiac surgery: rate of recovery and sequelae. Otolaryngol Head Neck Surg 2007;137(5):780–4.

49. Joo D, Duarte VM, Ghadiali MT, et al. Recovery of vocal fold paralysis after cardiovascular surgery. Laryngoscope 2009;119(7):1435–8.

50. Brigger MT, Hartnick CJ. Surgery for pediatric vocal cord paralysis: a meta-analysis. Otolaryngol Head Neck Surg 2002;126:349–55.

51. Ossoff RH, Sisson GA, Duncavage JA, et al. Endoscopic laser arytenoidectomy for the treatment of bilateral vocal cord paralysis. Laryngoscope 1984;94:1293–7.

52. Dennis DP, Kashima H. Carbon dioxide laser posterior cordectomy for treatment of bilateral vocal cord paralysis. Ann Otol Rhinol Laryngol 1989;98:930–4.

53. Bizakis JG, Papadakis CE, Karatzanis AD, et al. The combined endoscopic CO(2) laser posterior cordectomy and total arytenoidectomy for treatment of bilateral vocal cord paralysis. Clin Otolaryngol Allied Sci 2004;29:51–4.

54. Friedman EM, de Jong AL, Sulek M. Pediatric bilateral vocal fold immobility: the role of carbon dioxide laser posterior transverse partial cordectomy. Ann Otol Rhinol Laryngol 2001;110:723–8.

55. Mathur NN, Kumar S, Bothra R. Simple method of vocal cord lateralization in bilateral abductor cord paralysis in pediatric patients. Int J Pediatr Otorhinolaryngol 2004;68:15–20.

56. Rutter MJ, Hart CK, Alarcon A, et al. Endoscopic anterior-posterior cricoid split for pediatric bilateral vocal fold paralysis. Laryngoscope 2018;128(1):257–63.

57. Benjamin B, Inglis A. Minor congenital laryngeal clefts: diagnosis and classification. Ann Otol Rhinol Laryngol 1989;98(6):417–20.

58. Strychowsky JE, Dodrill P, Moritz E, et al. Swallowing dysfunction among patients with laryngeal cleft: more than just aspiration? Int J Pediatr Otorhinolaryngol 2016;82:38–42.

59. Chien W, Ashland J, Haver K, et al. Type I laryngeal cleft: establishing a functional diagnostic and management algorithm. Int J Pediatr Otorhinolaryngol 2006;70:2073–9.

60. Yoo MJ, Roy S, Smith LP. Endoscopic management of congenital anterior glottis stenosis. Int J Pediatr Otorhinolaryngol 2015;79(12):2056–8.

61. Rahbar R, Chen JL, Rosen RL, et al. Endoscopic repair of laryngeal cleft type I and type II: when and why? Laryngoscope 2009;119(9):1797–802.

62. Manickavasagam J, Yapa S, Bateman ND, et al. Congenital familial subglottic stenosis: a case series and review of literature. Int J Pediatr Otorhinolaryngol 2014;78(2):359–62.
63. Schroeder JW Jr, Holinger LD. Congenital laryngeal stenosis. Otolaryngol Clin North Am 2008;41(5):865–75.
64. Holinger LD. Histopathology of congenital subglottic stenosis. Ann Otol Rhinol Laryngol 1999;108:101–11.
65. Ferguson CF, Flake CG. Subglottic haemangioma as a cause of respiratory obstruction in infants. Ann Otol Rhinol Laryngol 1961;70:1095–112.
66. Bitar MA, Moukarbel RV, Zalzal GH. Management of congenital subglottic hemangioma: trends over the past 17 years. Otolaryngol Head Neck Surg 2005;132: 226–31.
67. Celiksoy MH, Paksu MS, Atmaca S, et al. Management of subglottic hemangioma with propranolol. Am J Otolaryngol 2014;35(3):414–6.
68. Li XY, Wang Y, Jin L, et al. Role of oral propranolol in the treatment of infantile subglottic hemangioma. Int J Clin Pharmacol Ther 2016;54(9):675–81.
69. Wang CF, Wang YS, Sun YF. Treatment of infantile subglottic hemangioma with oral propranolol. Pediatr Int 2016;58(5):385–8.
70. Rosbe KW, Suh KY, Meyer AK, et al. Propranolol in the management of airway infantile hemangiomas. Arch Otolaryngol Head Neck Surg 2010;136(7):658–65.
71. Raol N, Metry D, Edmonds J, et al. Propranolol for the treatment of subglottic hemangiomas. Int J Pediatr Otorhinolaryngol 2011;75(12):1510–4.
72. Hardison S, Wan W, Dodson KM. The use of propranolol in the treatment of subglottic hemangiomas: a literature review and meta-analysis. Int J Pediatr Otorhinolaryngol 2016;90:175–80.
73. Siegel B, Mehta D. Open airway surgery for subglottic hemangioma in the era of propranolol: is it still indicated? Int J Pediatr Otorhinolaryngol 2015;79(7):1124–7.
74. Usui N, Kamata S, Ishikawa S, et al. Anomalies of the tracheobronchial tree in patients with esophageal atresia. J Pediatr Surg 1996;31:258–62.
75. Malone PS, Kiely EM. Role of aortopexy in the management of primary tracheomalacia and tracheobronchomalacia. Arch Dis Child 1990;65:438–40.
76. Corbally MT, Spitz L, Kiely E, et al. Aortopexy for tracheomalacia in oesophageal anomalies. Eur J Pediatr Surg 1993;3:264–6.
77. Rutter MJ, Willging JP, Cotton RT. Nonoperative management of complete tracheal rings. Arch Otolaryngol Head Neck Surg 2004;130(4):450–2.
78. Elliot M, Roebuck D, Noctor C, et al. The management of congenital tracheal stenosis. Int J Pediatr Otorhinolaryngol 2003;67(suppl 1):S183–92.
79. Hofferberth SC, Watters K, Rahbar R, et al. Management of congenital tracheal stenosis. Pediatrics 2015;136(3):e660–9.

UNITED STATES POSTAL SERVICE® Statement of Ownership, Management, and Circulation (All Periodicals Publications Except Requester Publications)

1. Publication Title	2. Publication Number	3. Filing Date
CLINICS IN PERINATOLOGY	001 – 744	9/18/2018

4. Issue Frequency	5. Number of Issues Published Annually	6. Annual Subscription Price
MAR, JUN, SEP, DEC	4	$299.00

7. Complete Mailing Address of Known Office of Publication (Not printer) (Street, city, county, state, and ZIP+4®)

ELSEVIER INC.
230 Park Avenue, Suite 800
New York, NY 10169

Contact Person: STEPHEN R. BUSHING
Telephone (Include area code): 215-239-3688

8. Complete Mailing Address of Headquarters or General Business Office of Publisher (Not printer)

ELSEVIER INC.
230 Park Avenue, Suite 800
New York, NY 10169

9. Full Names and Complete Mailing Addresses of Publisher, Editor, and Managing Editor (Do not leave blank)

Publisher (Name and complete mailing address)
TAYLOR E BALL, ELSEVIER INC.
1600 JOHN F KENNEDY BLVD. SUITE 1800
PHILADELPHIA, PA 19103-2899

Editor (Name and complete mailing address)
KERRY HOLLAND, ELSEVIER INC.
1600 JOHN F KENNEDY BLVD. SUITE 1800
PHILADELPHIA, PA 19103-2899

Managing Editor (Name and complete mailing address)
PATRICK MANLEY, ELSEVIER INC.
1600 JOHN F KENNEDY BLVD. SUITE 1800
PHILADELPHIA, PA 19103-2899

10. Owner (Do not leave blank. If the publication is owned by a corporation, give the name and address of the corporation immediately followed by the names and addresses of all stockholders owning or holding 1 percent or more of the total amount of stock. If not owned by a corporation, give the names and addresses of the individual owners. If owned by a partnership or other unincorporated firm, give its name and address as well as those of each individual owner. If the publication is published by a nonprofit organization, give its name and address.)

Full Name	Complete Mailing Address
WHOLLY OWNED SUBSIDIARY OF REED/ELSEVIER, US HOLDINGS	1600 JOHN F KENNEDY BLVD. SUITE 1800 PHILADELPHIA, PA 19103-2899

11. Known Bondholders, Mortgagees, and Other Security Holders Owning or Holding 1 Percent or More of Total Amount of Bonds, Mortgages, or Other Securities. If none, check box ▶ ☒ None

Full Name	Complete Mailing Address
N/A	

12. Tax Status (For completion by nonprofit organizations authorized to mail at nonprofit rates) (Check one)
The purpose, function, and nonprofit status of this organization and the exempt status for federal income tax purposes:
☒ Has Not Changed During Preceding 12 Months
☐ Has Changed During Preceding 12 Months (Publisher must submit explanation of change with this statement)

PS Form 3526, July 2014 [Page 1 of 4 (see instructions page 4)] PSN: 7530-01-000-9931   PRIVACY NOTICE: See our privacy policy on www.usps.com.

---

13. Publication Title	14. Issue Date for Circulation Data Below
CLINICS IN PERINATOLOGY	JUNE 2018

15. Extent and Nature of Circulation		Average No. Copies Each Issue During Preceding 12 Months	No. Copies of Single Issue Published Nearest to Filing Date
a. Total Number of Copies (Net press run)		626	756
b. Paid Circulation (By Mail and Outside the Mail)	(1) Mailed Outside-County Paid Subscriptions Stated on PS Form 3541 (Include paid distribution above nominal rate, advertiser's proof copies, and exchange copies)	456	540
	(2) Mailed In-County Paid Subscriptions Stated on PS Form 3541 (Include paid distribution above nominal rate, advertiser's proof copies, and exchange copies)	0	0
	(3) Paid Distribution Outside the Mails Including Sales Through Dealers and Carriers, Street Vendors, Counter Sales, and Other Paid Distribution Outside USPS®	108	130
	(4) Paid Distribution by Other Classes of Mail Through the USPS (e.g., First-Class Mail®)	0	0
c. Total Paid Distribution (Sum of 15b (1), (2), (3), and (4))	▶	564	670
d. Free or Nominal Rate Distribution (By Mail and Outside the Mail)	(1) Free or Nominal Rate Outside-County Copies included on PS Form 3541	49	68
	(2) Free or Nominal Rate In-County Copies Included on PS Form 3541	0	0
	(3) Free or Nominal Rate Copies Mailed at Other Classes Through the USPS (e.g., First-Class Mail)	0	0
	(4) Free or Nominal Rate Distribution Outside the Mail (Carriers or other means)	0	0
e. Total Free or Nominal Rate Distribution (Sum of 15d (1), (2), (3) and (4))	▶	49	68
f. Total Distribution (Sum of 15c and 15e)	▶	613	738
g. Copies not Distributed (See Instructions to Publishers #4 (page 3))	▶	13	18
h. Total (Sum of 15f and g)	▶	626	756
i. Percent Paid (15c divided by 15f times 100)		92.01%	90.79%

* If you are claiming electronic copies, go to line 16 on page 3. If you are not claiming electronic copies, skip to line 17 on page 3.

16. Electronic Copy Circulation		Average No. Copies Each Issue During Preceding 12 Months	No. Copies of Single Issue Published Nearest to Filing Date
a. Paid Electronic Copies	▶	0	0
b. Total Paid Print Copies (Line 15c) + Paid Electronic Copies (Line 16a)	▶	564	670
c. Total Print Distribution (Line 15f) + Paid Electronic Copies (Line 16a)	▶	613	738
d. Percent Paid (Both Print & Electronic Copies) (16b divided by 16c × 100)	▶	92.01%	90.79%

☒ I certify that 50% of all my distributed copies (electronic and print) are paid above a nominal price.

17. Publication of Statement of Ownership
☒ If the publication is a general publication, publication of this statement is required. Will be printed in the DECEMBER 2018 issue of this publication.
☐ Publication not required.

18. Signature and Title of Editor, Publisher, Business Manager, or Owner

STEPHEN R. BUSHING - INVENTORY DISTRIBUTION CONTROL MANAGER

Date: 9/18/2018

I certify that all information furnished on this form is true and complete. I understand that anyone who furnishes false or misleading information on this form or who omits material or information requested on the form may be subject to criminal sanctions (including fines and imprisonment) and/or civil sanctions (including civil penalties).

PS Form 3526, July 2014 (Page 3 of 4)   PRIVACY NOTICE: See our privacy policy on www.usps.com

Moving?

Make sure your subscription moves with you!

To notify us of your new address, find your **Clinics Account Number** (located on your mailing label above your name), and contact customer service at:

Email: journalscustomerservice-usa@elsevier.com

800-654-2452 (subscribers in the U.S. & Canada)
314-447-8871 (subscribers outside of the U.S. & Canada)

Fax number: 314-447-8029

Elsevier Health Sciences Division
Subscription Customer Service
3251 Riverport Lane
Maryland Heights, MO 63043

*To ensure uninterrupted delivery of your subscription, please notify us at least 4 weeks in advance of move.

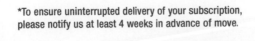